THE MENOPAUSE CURE:
HORMONAL HEALTH

THE MENOPAUSE CURE: HORMONAL HEALTH

By Jill D. Davey
With Sergey A. Dzugan MD PhD

Matador
9 Priory Business Park,
Wistow Road, Kibworth Beauchamp,
Leicestershire. LE8 0RX
Tel: 0116 279 2299
Email: books@troubador.co.uk
Web: www.troubador.co.uk/matador

ISBN 978 1784623 753

British Library Cataloguing in Publication Data.
A catalogue record for this book is available from the British Library.

Printed and bound by CPI Group (UK) Ltd, Croydon, CR0 4YY
Typeset by Troubador Publishing Ltd, Leicester, UK

Matador is an imprint of Troubador Publishing Ltd

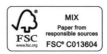

This book is dedicated to my parents, who are no longer with us, for making me the person I am today. I could not have asked more of them, or for better parents. They were always an inspiration to me, and without their guidance and encouragement, I could never have gone as far as I have. Thank you Mum and Dad, I love and miss you more with every day that passes.

Restorative medicine is an evidence-based, scientifically sound medical sub-speciality. Its goal is to extend lifespan, and prolong youthspan and healthspan through early detection, prevention, treatment and reversal of age-related dysfunction, disorders and diseases, in both men and women. It has been embraced by thousands of physicians.

Sergey A. Dzugan, MD, PhD, is co-founder and Chief Scientific Officer of the Dzugan Institute of Restorative Medicine, Deerfield Beach, Fl. and co-founder of DzLogic inc., and a former heart surgeon. The International Academy of Creative Endeavors (Russia) awarded Dr Dzugan the honorary title of Academician for his outstanding contribution to the development of new methods of hypercholesterolemia and migraine treatment. He has delivered multiple presentations at the prestigious International Congress on Anti-Ageing Medicine. He is the author of five books, 151 publications in medical journals and numerous articles in health-related magazines, and holds three patents. Dr Dzugan is a member of the Editorial Board of *Neuroendocrinology Letters*, and of the Medical Advisory Board at *Life Extension Magazine*. He is co-founder and President of iPOMS (International Physiology Optimization Medical Society).

CONTENTS

FOREWORD

You've perhaps heard the horror stories that make you dread that pivotal life moment, or even experienced its symptoms. At some point, you possibly succumbed to the idea that menopause or aging itself meant losing your libido, waistline and *joie de vivre* as you reluctantly surrender to its merciless repercussions.

I'm here to tell you that with the right approach, menopause and the years surrounding it can become the most amazing time in your life. Having the right tools and strategies can transform this life transition into a self-awakening and even spiritual experience.

That's where *The Menopause Cure* can become your trusted best friend, if your best friend just happens to be a knowledgeable, savvy medical doctor, such as Dr Sergey Dzugan.

In this groundbreaking, informative book, Jill Davey and Dr Sergey Dzugan dive deep into hormones, potential complications and symptoms, troubleshooting without becoming encyclopaedic or pedantic.

Restorative medicine becomes the foundation of their approach. Unlike conventional medicine, restorative medicine treats the body as a wondrous, intricately connected organism composed of an amazing hormonal team. When your hormones perform optimally you feel vibrant, exuberant and sexy. Fast, lasting fat loss becomes attainable. You joyously embrace growing older with confidence and zeal.

Unfortunately, our fast-faster, super-hectic lives mean many of us suffer out-of-whack hormones, with all their consequences. We get too little sleep, struggle with chronic stress, over-exercise (or more likely, don't exercise at all) and graze on a high-sugar impact diet. Like an unruly employee who can wreck your whole team's morale, one out-of-whack hormone creates a vicious domino effect with disastrous repercussions. Take insulin. When this fat-storing hormone becomes out of balance, other hormones quickly follow. Your stress hormone, cortisol, stays elevated when it should taper down, your thyroid crashes, your satiety hormone, leptin, stops communicating with your brain (called leptin resistance), and so you suddenly discover yourself mindlessly devouring a double fudge brownie, and your sex hormones take a massive nosedive.

It isn't your fault you struggle with weight loss resistance, crave sugar, have zero sex drive and constantly feel as if you're running on empty. Your hormones have become messed up, and *The Menopause Cure* provides the blueprint to fix them.

There are no quick solutions here, but once you're in the driver's seat you can correct these imbalances. When you do, you'll discover that you're not struggling with mid-afternoon doughnut cravings, and you'll finally lose weight, and feel sexy, radiant and confident.

I've witnessed this transformation with colleagues, friends, family, and in my own life. Whereas we once dreaded the M word, today we thrive into midlife and beyond. We feel fabulous, stay lean and muscular, have more energy than women half our age, and – yeah, I'll say it – enjoy the most amazing sex of our lives.

Armed with this information, you'll have a complete understanding of how hormones perform and interact. You'll have an arsenal of strategies if you experience the complications of menopause, and you'll be able to have an intelligent conversation with your healthcare professional about topics like bio-identical hormones.

The Menopause Cure ultimately becomes a self-investing guide to reclaim your health. "We do not have to follow the old

template of ageing and conventional medical care," writes Jill
Davey, "We have a choice; why not take it?"

You needn't succumb to weight gain, fuzzy thinking,
diminishing libido and other menopause-related symptoms.
Here's to reclaiming your life and gracefully embracing health,
happiness and joy!

J. J. Virgin

www.jjvirgin.com

Author of *The Sugar Impact Diet* and *The Virgin Diet*

PREFACE

In the past I have written books that focused on the aging problem, but always from the viewpoint of the physician, which presented issues with relatability. There are many books on this topic, but the majority of them were written by medical doctors. Now you have the opportunity to read a beautifully written book about female issues related to aging from the viewpoint of both a patient and a layperson.

Many difficult problems are presented in a simple and easy-to-understand way, but are well backed up with the proper scientific data. Jill masterfully examines the core of various issues using a basis in scientific analysis while still presenting the information in a very understandable way. She writes not only about the problems, but also their origin, which allows for a discussion about preventative measures without resorting to drugs and their side effects. A point is made regarding solving issues via a physiological approach, an approach that is described as being fully grounded in the study of how the body functions on a daily basis.

During the progress of aging the body no longer works in an optimal way. This entire process is relatively complex, and breaking it down adequately for comprehension is not an easy task. In this case, however, this task is very well executed.

I want to applaud Jill for the terrific job she's done. I hope that you will enjoy reading this book and take full advantage of the wealth of information contained within it.

Dr Dzugan
Founder and Director
DZLogic

ACKNOWLEDGEMENTS

I could not have written this book if it were not for Dr Sergey Dzugan. He listened to me when I spoke and when I asked questions, he answered them without hesitation. He gave me the opportunity and the information I desired to inspire, educate and join hands with women throughout the Western world, to let them know that menopause does not have to be the end of life as we know it today, but a rebirth, a new beginning. Thank you Dr Dzugan for your assistance in the writing of this book – you taught me so much, and I am deeply indebted to you. Thank you for your time and inexhaustible knowledge. What a fantastic doctor to work with.

Thank you to my husband, Giorgio, and my two grown-up sons, Jonathan and Joshua, for their support, enthusiasm and for believing in me, enabling me to sit in the 'driver's seat' once again. Thank you Giorgio for listening to me when I needed someone to explain things to, and thank you for loving me, giving me the confidence that has empowered me to attain my highest goals.

Thank you Dianne, my dear and lifelong friend, who never lets me down. Who encouraged me to write this book. Who believed in me. Thank you Dianne for being there when I most needed you. Thank you for reading *The Menopause Cure*, and giving me your thoughts and opinions.

INTRODUCTION

The majority of you reading this book will be women who are either entering menopause (perimenopause), or who have been through menopause and have come out on the other side of the tracks. You are probably feeling, or have felt, the changes that have taken place in your body, leaving you a totally different person, both mentally and physically. You are holding this book in your hands because you are curious to know how restorative medicine can guide you through, over, and beyond this inevitable passage of time and out into a world you never knew existed. Back into that world from which you came. One of happiness, vitality, energy, mental clarity, productivity, youthfulness, strength, and screaming positivity. These are some of the things I lost in perimenopause; I lost my edge, but reclaimed it when I restored my body. I now have the best of both worlds. You can too – restorative medicine can give you all of this, and you can have the worldly knowledge of a mature woman together with the youth and vitality of a twenty-five-year-old. How's that for trumps? And importantly, you can have back the 'you' you once were. So many women lose their confidence, self-esteem, sensuality, creativity and energy in this phase of their lives. I know I certainly couldn't have written this book, or been the person I am today, had I not embraced this medicine.

Restorative medicine is a new medicine: a real medicine. This is a branch of medicine that strengthens the immune system and builds the body back up, balancing hormones with the use of natural, bioidentical hormones. A medicine that maintains the balance within the body and its systems, and offers us an amazing opportunity to live a long, healthy, disease-free life. We have become used to accepting ageing and the menopause as a normal process. Accepting getting fat, a diminished sex drive, suffering hot flushes and night sweats, being unable to sleep peacefully anymore, sudden brain fog and senior moments that, at times, can be so embarrassing. Accepting becoming ill, feeble, weak and depressed; disinterested in life. Accepting down-beaten-hearts and heart disease, high blood pressure, diabetes, osteoporosis, dementia and more. We do not have to accept this anymore. There is an alternative, a safe method to redress all menopausal symptoms, and the disease they now call ageing, along with all of its age-related diseases. Life truly can begin again at fifty (and after). I am here for you, together with Dr Dzugan, to act as an 'information point', and to introduce you to this new approach to medicine. I want to tweak your curiosity, open your eyes, help you understand that restorative medicine is the name of the game. I want you to start loving yourselves, caring about yourselves; I want you to start investigating this cutting-edge medicine that wants to treat you and allow you to be healthy and prevent you getting ill, not wait until your body is so broken and sick it can no longer be treated.

This book discusses menopause in depth, a phase in life women cannot avoid; the other side of life. Life isn't as much fun as it used to be. Women are so used to being told, "It's only the menopause, it'll pass." Totally untrue. Yes, your hot flushes and night sweats will pass but internally the body is experiencing total breakdown due to hormonal loss. It doesn't pass, it gets worse. This is why we become weak, frail, have bent-up bodies and get sick as we age. The major part of it is to do with hormonal loss. Hot flushes are transitory, they are a symptom telling our body that something is not functioning correctly; something has gone awry. Transitory because they apparently pass, they last only as long as it takes for the body to adapt to this new situation. This new situation is dangerous and will eventually lead to chronic disease and ageing, so it needs to be corrected. Declining hormones need to be restored for the body to function optimally, and to slow the 'body breakdown' process. Hormones have an incredible influence on the body – they control us, they make or break us, build us up or tear us down. With declining hormone levels we age at a greater rate, and die at a greater speed.

Hormones guide the body; they are a go-between, a messenger communicating between the cells, expertly talking to them and telling them what to do. When hormones decline the message is not fully received and the body shifts into a state of imbalance. We cannot think straight anymore, weight goes up for no apparent reason, sexuality drops to levels never felt before, skin becomes sallow, saggy and wrinkles out of control. We can't cope as well as we once did, hair loses its full-bodied shine and lustre, eyesight starts to fade, and regulating body temperature becomes impossible. With balanced hormones these symptoms go away. With declining hormones we are slowly fading away and towards an uncomfortable old age. Again, we have become used to accepting that dying of cancer, heart disease and Alzheimer's, the three major killers, is the norm. It doesn't have to be; this is the 'old approach'. This is not the way we have to age, live and die.

By restoring your hormones, and making lifestyle adjustments, which include healthy eating, stress reduction, detoxification and regular exercise, we can look forward to a fantastic old age, full of vitality, energy, sex drive, a fully functioning brain, and health. This applies to both men and women. When I talk about hormones, I don't mean the synthetic type produced by the pharmaceutical industries, I mean bioidentical hormones, natural hormones. Synthetic hormones are dangerous – I will discuss this in more depth in the book. It is up to you to take charge of your life. You are on your own. No one else can take care of you as you do yourself. This book helps you to understand how your body works, and teaches you that everything in the body is interconnected. It is a step-by-step guide. I feel that it is important for you to be informed, as only then can you truly begin to look forward to the second half of your life. This 'new medicine', cutting-edge medicine, offers you the most forward approach to combating illness and disability. It offers you life.

It is quite clear that the 'old school approach' to medicine is inefficient – it doesn't work. Yes, conventional medicine, together with technology, has given us the possibility to live longer but quality of life is just not there. Is that what you really want? Are you ready for those gruelling last years of discomfort and pain, hanging on? Restorative medicine, the 'new school approach', works. It gives us both longevity and health.

What this book does is to teach you how to thrive and survive in old age. You will learn how to avoid cancer, how to normalise cholesterol levels naturally, without the use of statin drugs, and how to overcome migraines. You will learn how to achieve balanced hormones at optimal levels. Restorative medicine's objective is to be healthy from the inside out. You will learn about the minor and major hormones; you will learn about the sex hormones, progesterone, oestrogens and testosterone, and about all the other hormones that are key to your health, and how they function within the body. You will learn about the dangers of perimenopause and how to avoid these dangers. Perimenopause is a transition that is little understood, both by doctors and the woman who is going through it. This book will explain why it is important to pay attention to your health at this stage in your life. You will learn about what happens to the body during menopause and after menopause. You will learn how to correct, slow and, in some cases, reverse the ageing process. You will learn how to expand your youthspan and how to live a long, healthy, disease-free life. You will learn not to fear those coming years because you don't have to fear getting old.

This medicine is for everyone. Men are not as proactive about their health as women, but declining hormone levels affect them just as much. They too lose their sex drive, vitality, sharp thinking and muscle. They too have to face those terrible age-related diseases. The ageing process affects them just as much. There is no getting away from it – cancer, weight gain, muscle loss, diabetes, osteoporosis, heart disease and dementia. These things are all related to declining hormones. Men too can restore their body and avoid these age-related diseases.

Restorative medicine is a very precise medicine that requires intricate blood tests. We are all different and therefore require different supplements in different amounts. Once your blood samples are analysed, you will then be prescribed bioidentical hormones, supplements, vitamins and minerals based on where your optimal levels should be. If your blood tests show that you are low on magnesium, calcium or iron you will be prescribed whichever is needed to bring you within optimal ranges. Another example is that if you are low on the two female sex hormones, progesterone and oestrogens, they will be prescribed, within their required ratios, again to bring you within optimal ranges. Bioidentical hormones, vitamins, supplements and minerals work together in the body; they are all interrelated. As Dr Dzugan said to me, "Your blood doesn't lie, it is not guesswork – this is a precise medicine. Your bloodwork shows what is missing and what is needed at that time. This medicine tells you what your body needs and what it doesn't need."

Going into a pharmacy and haphazardly picking up vitamins and minerals off the shelf is not a part of restorative medicine's philosophy. It is all based on bloodwork; this is not a one-size-fits-all medicine. I know what I am putting into my body. I am balanced and I feel good.

1. LET'S STEP INTO MY LIFE

The Beginning of the Beginning of the Second Half of My Life

Saturday mornings were something I looked forward to. They were reserved for cappuccino with friends at Bar Centrale in Riccione Paese, an old northern Italian town. It was a tradition but lately things had become kind of different. Suddenly things had changed; things had crept up on us before we'd realised. There wasn't a time in our fun-loving meetings that I didn't hear about some friend or other who'd been diagnosed with cancer – breast cancer was a biggie – or someone who had high blood pressure, high cholesterol, diabetes, fibromyalgia, heart disease, depression and even Alzheimer's – nearly everyone's parents seemed to have it, if not their auntie or uncle. Along with breast cancer, the words 'weight gain' and 'migraine' started appearing in our vocabulary. Must be to do with the menopause, was the consensus. The list goes on and on. And you men, you do not stand to attention anymore: erectile dysfunction, prostate problems, drop-dead heart attacks. So what's going on? There is a common denominator. These are all things that come with age. This is called a diseased state, when the body is not functioning correctly. This is a breakdown of physiologic function. These are acquired physiological errors, as Dr Dzugan explains it.

The Declining Hormone Phenomenon

And my decline didn't get any better. It brought with it changes I didn't understand; every day of the week there was something: mood swings, lack of energy, 'can't cope' syndrome, grumpy, general unhappiness. A personality change had occurred and I really didn't like myself anymore. I couldn't sleep peacefully anymore, and I was tearing my hair out. Help!

Waking up sluggish was not a good feeling, especially when six months previously, I had been waking up at 6am to go running along the beach. Even pulling myself out of bed at 8am became a problem. Taking an hour and a half to come round in the morning was not a good feeling either – I was later to find out that I had a condition called subclinical hypothyroidism. And sex: what's that? Uncomfortable and painful; didn't want it anymore. Even my memory was in decline – I kept forgetting the simplest of things, and even lost my car one day. When I found it again I managed to bump into the back of the car in front. I was distracted, couldn't concentrate. Multitasking became difficult. What was happening? That just wasn't me. And goodness, that mirror every morning, not a happy place to be! Tired, haggard and drawn; every day there was something: patchy, dry, red skin on my face or one more wrinkle around my eyes to add to the list. Was that really me? I was ageing fast. I'd always had such a good skin. I decided to take the magnifying mirror off the wall. Who dared look so close?

What an age fifty was. Like I said, a personality change had occurred, and my body was in 'breakdown' mode. I don't necessarily mean that I was ill but I certainly was not the me I had once been. This strange being had taken over me a few years previously, at forty-six. I was someone I couldn't handle anymore, someone I didn't know and didn't like. I started getting more infections, colds and flu too, which meant courses of antibiotics. I had always been such a well person. In fact, people used to ask me how come I never got flu. My answer was, "I look after myself and eat well. (Our food is our fuel. We truly are what we eat. Food builds us up or pulls us down.) I exercise, I've never smoked and I keep wine to a minimum, maybe three glasses a week." Good Italian wine that comes from our small family vineyard, and pure cold-pressed olive oil from our olive trees. I drizzle this on my home-grown organic salad daily.

I very rarely took pharmaceuticals unless really necessary, and never ever took the contraceptive pill long-term. Of course, that is maybe why I got pregnant five times – so much for the safe method. Luckily for me, I couldn't take the pill; it made me feel ill, not quite right. After just one month of taking the contraceptive pill I felt strange, uneasy. It just didn't connect with my body. I am very sensitive, and my body seems to know what it wants and does not want. By the way, and unfortunately, I did not have five children, I only have two wonderful boys, now aged eighteen and twenty-three. Sadly, I miscarried with the other three, not a good time for me. Had I only known about restorative medicine, I could have avoided those miscarriages. It was my hormones – they were all mixed up and there was an imbalance. When there is optimal balance and optimal levels of basic hormones such as progesterone, oestrogens and DHEA, it decreases the risk of a miscarriage. Something was amiss.

At fifty-one, the situation got worse. I was even more sad and tired, I was breathless, bitchy and itchy, bloated and sore-throated. Sex was out of the window for good, or so I thought! And those night sweats – waking up drenched in sweat, at first I actually thought I had a temperature. Then my skin broke out and my eyes started to water: an allergy had arrived on my doorstep. As far as I was concerned, I was definitely not menopausal and that was that; I was far too young and anyway, the menopause just didn't happen like that! But of course it did, and I was.

This was the time in my life when I really woke up. It was like a slap on the face: why hadn't someone warned me about this? I had glided through life without a care in the world. Everything had always been great for me. I'd always made it go great for me – a great family life, wonderful husband, a successful business. I was invincible, or at least I thought I was. Then suddenly, there I was, in the MENOPAUSE and unable to cope – things were going wrong. In my books that meant I was old, and depression hit me. That meant that I could only look forward to doom and gloom. Oh no, no, not for me! I remembered my mother and her personality change too. I remembered her hysterectomy, her general decline in quality of life and everything else that supposedly goes with the menopause. She battled through it all on her own – hot flushes, mood swings and all – while at the same time taking care of three teenage children (me, my twin brother and elder sister by two years) and her own mother, as well as a full-time job to juggle with. How difficult it must have been for her, and no one understood. I certainly didn't understand at the time. I do now though.

I was determined my voyage into menopause, and beyond, would be a positive one; let's face it, it's something we cannot avoid. I decided that I had to make this inevitable destiny an enjoyable one. I went to many doctors and gynaecologists to find a solution, but to no avail. All I got was a mixture of anger and ignorance. My anger and their ignorance.

My anger, because I refused to be this person I had become: negative and not so pleasant. Sniffing and coughing all the way. My anger, because I refused to accept that these doctors I was searching out were waving me out of their office and telling me, "It's only the menopause, and not to worry, it'll pass." What were they on about? Angry, because I was in the menopause and I couldn't believe it – I was far too young, and it just seemed to happen overnight. Angry because apparently I couldn't do anything about it except play the waiting game.

Their ignorance, that wave of the hand in sharp dismissal; menopause, menopause, menopause, over and over again. Their ignorance, a lack of desire to help. "Look at me, I am begging you, help me!" All they could do was hand out a few medicines, antibiotics, antidepressants and HRT, which in their minds would solve the problem. Now, why on earth would I want to take a pill (HRT) that was produced from horses' urine and contains various potent oestrogens, one of which is equilin? This may be fine for a horse but we are humans, or did someone forget something? And why would I take a pill that was going to mess with my body and most likely provoke cancer? Would I drink the stuff?

I am a mover and I always move forward. I am a thinker and I always think positively, hard and long. There is always something better we can get from life whatever our age. Positivity and determination create success, it doesn't just happen. You create the pathway to success. Success is connected to health; you cannot be successful if you are not healthy, either in life or in business.

To make matters even worse, my sister was diagnosed with breast cancer for the second time while I was going through the trials and tribulations of menopause and my body and mind breaking down. She was forty-seven when first diagnosed with breast cancer. Why, why, why? Why did she get cancer? Were her hormones out of whack or was it the fact that she had been exposed to DES (diethylstilbestrol) *in utero*? (We will talk about DES later.) These questions came to me over and over again. My poor sister. A life-changing experience.

Changing of the Guards!

This is when I decided things had to change. There had to be something out there in this modern world that could get me through this, and perhaps help my sister as well.

I immersed myself in research, which was quite bland in the beginning, but as the passion grew, my research became more extensive, more intensive and more and more expensive. I kept reading about bioidentical hormones and restorative medicine. Bioidentical hormones can help prevent cancer. Bioidentical hormones can slow down the disease they now call ageing. Bioidentical hormones can prevent heart attacks and strokes, high cholesterol, osteoporosis… the list went on and on. I started attending conferences around the world, listening and almost grappling for information. I got the opportunity to speak with these highly qualified anti-ageing doctors. They welcomed a layperson asking questions and were very receptive towards my curiosity. Talking to these doctors is incredible. The knowledge they hold is inexhaustible, very powerful and cutting-edge science. One of these doctors was Dr Sergey Dzugan, co-founder of Dzugan PhysioLogic. He is considered a world-renowned expert in physiology and hormonal restorative medicine. He found a cure for migraine that really works, and a method for normalising cholesterol levels by optimising body physiology. No nasty pharmaceutical drugs involved.

Dr Dzugan is my teacher, as I hope he will become yours. He has so much to teach us, so many clearly explained hypotheses, which will follow in the next chapters, but first we need to know how the body works, and how we function. From that we can begin to understand. Have you ever asked yourself why the body slows and stops working with age, or do you just accept it? It's the 'common denominator'.

Have you ever asked yourself if your hormonal glands are functioning or dysfunctioning? Do you know anything about hormones or glands, the endocrine system, the immune system, your gut, the sympathetic or parasympathetic nervous systems, your HPA (hypothalamus, pituitary and adrenal) axis, or your body in general for that matter? Parasites. Dr Dzugan keeps talking about parasites. Yuk! Parasites in my body? No way. Can you imagine having those awful creatures squirming around in your body? They have no place there. Human parasites such as protozoa and worms need to stay away from us, a long way away. These parasites are picked up easily through the food chain, through water and, without doubt, through travelling. So many people travel these days and don't even realise they come home with these parasites in their digestive tract, which can cause inflammation. Get those parasites out of my GI tract, out of my body.

Do you know anything about physiology? Well, neither did I until I asked Dr Dzugan to explain. Physiology simply refers to a normal, functioning, healthy body, with physiology itself being the science behind this. "Yeah," I said to myself, "of course I know what physiology is, well, the word anyway, but not the actual concept." Do you understand what restorative medicine is?

Am I Afraid of Getting Old?

I have asked myself many, many times if I'm afraid of getting old. Yes, of course I am, isn't everyone? I am afraid of getting age-related diseases such as Alzheimer's, macular degenerative disease, heart disease, cancer, diabetes, and of becoming feeble and weak, and depressed. No, that's not for me. Ooooh no! I love life. I know we all die and there is absolutely nothing we can do about it, but the possibility of restoring our body, keeping our cells healthy, restoring our energy, vitality, brain function, sexuality and vigour is, to me anyway, extremely exciting. This is how I want my old age to be: strong, vibrant, healthy, full of joy. I want to see my grandchildren and even my great-grandchildren; I want to be happy and connected when I play with them. This is possible! We can prevent these diseases ever happening, we can protect ourselves by making the right decisions. This is the secret to longevity and to a healthy mind and body. We can decide how we want to grow old. I am a true believer in restorative medicine. I know what it can do for you; I live with myself every day and know that the path I have taken is the correct one. This is a scientifically-based medicine that is sound and steadfast.

Ask yourself this question, as I have done many times. Where do you want to be in twenty or thirty years' time? Now sit down with a notepad and write down how you want your life to be. Write about how you see your life, where you want to be: in a wheelchair, an old people's home, or in your own home, standing in your kitchen, cooking your own food? In your own home sitting in your own armchair, or lying sick in hospital? Ask yourself. Visualise your life and where you will be: healthy in mind and body, independent and free, or locked up and isolated in your own little world, not remembering anything because of severe hormonal degradation. Write that list and plan your future life; that way you will see which way you want to go. I know where I am going.

Hormones are the essence of life. With the use of bioidentical hormones, vitamins and minerals, you can become truly well, like me. This is medicine that will save your life and make it worth living. Restorative medicine is cutting-edge medicine.

Yes, the essence of life. I can't say enough about bioidentical hormones; they have changed my life, my body, my mind, my being. This is the best I have ever felt – well, since I was thirty-five, at least. I am passionate about them. My individualised programme that is perfectly balanced has knocked menopause on the head. Even though I am ageing chronologically, I am 'holding back the years', staving off disease and restoring and maintaining internal youth and energy. Age is just a number that does not interest me anymore. I am continually astonished by my energy and am always asking myself how can I possibly be growing older, yet feeling younger? How can I have regained my love of dancing in the kitchen and listening to music? That is something I also lost with my personality change. Music became a noise to me, and I didn't like any noise, it irritated me. I needed peace and quiet. In my younger days I would dance in the kitchen while preparing dinner, Gloria Gaynor blaring out 'Never Can Say Goodbye'. This is my song; it's the song I play today. I can never say goodbye to bioidentical hormones, which are the backbone to restorative medicine. Once you have tasted the truths of restorative medicine you will never, ever let go. The amazing health benefits and sheer joy this medicine can give you is incredible. Jumping out of bed in the morning, feeling frisky and full of energy, drawing back the curtains with a smile on your face, eager to start the day – life is great and it's my birthday today, another year older. Who cares? I feel great.

Restorative medicine is the only thing that can ward off illness, fatigue, migraine, that debilitating life you had to live. Finally you have peace, no more explosions in your head, no more high cholesterol levels, no more weight gain and all the symptoms associated with hormonal decline. These hormones, bioidentical hormones, are life-giving hormones. With the use of restorative medicine you'll glide through the menopause and onwards, to a new lease of life.

Oh, and another thing: no more colds, flu or infections – an antibiotic-free life. And I do not want to get cancer. I have built my immune system up! Hormones are my love, my life, my energy.

Without a healthy immune system we cannot be truly well. When our hormones are balanced and our gut is functioning correctly, our immune system will be strong. The immune system declines with age, along with our hormones. A healthy immune system starts in the GI tract, accounting for 70% of our immunity. What we eat (junk food), antibiotics, pesticides, fluoride, chlorine, over-the-counter drugs, food intolerances and allergies all affect the function of the gut and when the gut becomes inflamed due to these continual assaults, the immune system downgrades. This is when the invader has a chance to get in. The immune system keeps us healthy, strong and fighting fit! Without a healthy GI tract we cannot have a healthy immune system and we certainly cannot keep those nasty parasites in their place. We cannot avoid getting a cold or flu. Have you ever asked yourself why some people catch colds and flu when others don't? The answer is in the strength of your immune system – is it working at an optimal level? We make the choices that strengthen or weaken our immune system. Our immune system is the protector of our health and vitality, which enables us to feel good both physically and emotionally. If our immune system is weak we are less able to handle stress and more susceptible to illnesses. When our immune system is suppressed over a long period, we are definitely more likely to suffer from far more serious diseases such as breast cancer, arthritis, autoimmune diseases and more. I am protecting my protector. Are you? A major component of having a strong immune system is restoring hormone levels.

Inflammation at its Best or at its Worst!

There are not many people, even doctors for that matter, who really understand inflammation. So, before I go any further with this incredible journey, I would like to discuss inflammation and its connection to chronic disease and the ageing process.

Inflammation is not just a cut on your finger that turns red, swells and feels hot, or a temperature due to an infection. There is more to inflammation than meets the eye. This kind of inflammation is our body working at its most basic level; it is our body's defence mechanism, its natural healing process against infection, toxins and injury. Our defence mechanism is set to immediately attack any lethal microbes that enter our body; this is the body's way of healing. The body needs a certain amount of inflammation to be healthy. If we do not have it, we cannot fight off infections and kill cancers. Inflammation is our body at work, it is an indication that pro-inflammatory chemicals (cytokines) in the blood are at work, disabling and healing tissue by way of repair. Thank goodness.

Unfortunately, as life would have it, inflammation is also linked to ageing and declining hormone levels. Ageing and a hormonal imbalance bring with them an inability to turn off inflammatory reactions, which creates an imbalance between destructive and protective inflammatory responses. This is what most people don't know or understand about inflammation. This imbalance creates low-level systemic inflammation that slowly destroys tissue by launching an attack on our normal cells. Our body is gradually shifting into a state of chronic inflammation, also known as inflammaging. Inflammation has now become the chronic form rather than the transitory form which is needed for our protection. You may not be able to see it, but it is there, lurking about inside you. If you have constant pain in your leg or arm, if you have a chronic cough, or are always clearing your chest or throat, if you suffer from chronic fatigue or chronic heartburn, these are all symptoms of what you may have to face later on. Inflammation is the body's way of talking to us; it is a message, a warning, and this is when we need to learn to listen.

Transitory inflammation can include sore throats, toothache, a sprained wrist or an oozing infection. Chronic inflammation is something deep-rooted. It is not good. It is dangerous. It is age-related, can be genetically related (but that does not mean we *have* to get it), or it can be related to the environment. If we insist on eating badly – an unhealthy diet full of bad fats, or a high glycaemic diet – and smoke, together with no exercise, it puts extra pressure on our body, which keeps the inflammatory process chugging along. A change of lifestyle will definitely help. Smoking is one of the factors that lead to plaque in the arteries, among other health problems. That is one definition of chronic inflammation. Chronic inflammation is also linked to conditions such as diabetes, cancer, rheumatoid arthritis, colitis, cardiovascular disease, Alzheimer's and digestive system diseases. Chronic inflammation attacks cells throughout our body, causing damage to our brain cells and the lining of our arteries, while about 25% of cancers are linked to chronic inflammation. Chronic inflammation harms us and is associated with nearly every age-related disease there is. It is the driving force behind these terrifying middle-and old-aged diseases we see every day.

What is even less understood is that at the same time, our immune system weakens, and so its response to pathological killers, the 'invader' microorganisms and abnormal cells, is diminished. This imbalance is an additional trigger to all diseases of ageing and an early grave. A loss of immune function leaves us wide open and vulnerable to all of these chronic diseases. Age is a terrible thing unless we at least try and control it. Age changes the way our body functions and the way our immune system functions, by increasing unwanted (inappropriate) inflammation and suppressing needed (appropriate) immune responses.

Chronic inflammation is serious business, so should be taken seriously. You need to catch inflammation in time before it catches you. Catch those major killers before they get you! Restorative medicine can help you get your body back on track, and/or keep it stable. Restorative medicine will help you understand where you are and help steer you off the pathway to chronic disease and an early death.

2. ARE YOU READY TO ROCK AND ROLL?

Restorative medicine is a complicated sector for the newcomer and needs to be understood in its entirety. Anyone hearing the words for the first time may be dubious, but the more you read this book, the more you will understand the workings of it and see how wonderful and, at the end of the day, logical it is. With this basic knowledge we can stride forward and truly become well; we can reach optimal health, as we had in our youth. Without this knowledge we cannot change, we cannot become well, we cannot jump for joy, we cannot stay physically, mentally and emotionally fit. We can only look forward to the three major age-related killers: cancer, heart disease and Alzheimer's, along with depression, macular degeneration, shattered bones (osteoporosis), arthritis and a sick, painful, uncomfortable old age. God forbid, don't let this happen.

Medicine today is at a turning point; things need to change. Restorative medicine is that change. People are asking questions, they want to know why, how, what and where. We need to look at science. This science shows us that we can get right down in there and treat the root cause rather than just the symptom.

Defining Restorative Medicine

Restorative medicine does exactly that: it gets to the root cause. Restorative medicine views our body and health in a complete sense – a whole-body approach. Being of optimal health is what we are looking at – being emotionally, mentally and spiritually connected, a ripple of water flowing smoothly and constantly. The hormonal network along with internal organs and systems functioning at maximum efficiency. Restorative medicine looks at prevention, not only cure, by keeping things in balance. The real goal is to restore function and not necessarily treat disease – this is the essence of restorative medicine. Restorative medicine is for everyone; we don't have to wait for the body to go into physiological breakdown mode before searching for a qualified restorative doctor.

Restorative medicine addresses the breakdown of physiological function and corrects physiological error, which we acquire with age, by optimising our physiological profile. One of the many things we achieve by optimising our health is to rebuild our immune system which helps us to avoid certain cancers. Remember, our immune system is a great part of what keeps us out of trouble, keeps us strong and healthy. With an inadequate immune system, the invader can easily attack. Hormones play the star role in optimising our physiological profile and also have an enormous influence on our immune system, amongst other things. Restorative medicine replaces what is missing, thereby restoring our body and physiological function.

At a basic level what I am saying is that restorative medicine corrects and balances instead of suppressing and hiding those niggling symptoms, which will, at a later date, become something 'not so very nice'. Symptoms are a warning sign; your body is talking to you. Restorative medicine does not move around in the mist, it focuses clearly on the symptom, identifies the underlying cause and corrects it. It focuses on YOU, the patient! The overall goal of restorative medicine is to prevent these symptoms ever occurring by keeping hormones balanced, synchronised, or let's say, in key, in harmony, with the use of bioidentical hormones, vitamins, supplements and minerals, all of which are important for a long and healthy life. Restorative medicine approaches the body with true health and prevention in mind. We need an in-depth knowledge of ourselves, both physically and mentally, before our health deteriorates to the point of no return, and to do this we need to become aware, to understand. Be aware of what is happening around us and within us.

Let's Take a Quick Look at the Other Side: Conventional Medicine

Conventional medicine views the body as being disease-free, physically healthy, until a symptom occurs. Conventional medicine waits for the symptom to appear rather than preventing it from ever happening. What happens next? Your doctor will look to treat the isolated symptom rather than the cause. Conventional medicine does not look deeper. Your doctor will diagnose whichever problem, be it heart (cardiology), a neurological disease (neurology), or a stomach problem (gastroenterology), etc., then in turn, will direct you to a specialist who will treat that particular symptom. You may be given an X-ray, a CT scan, a mammogram, a biopsy. These methods do not get to the root cause – they may find the symptom but they do not get to the bottom of where the symptom or symptoms is/are coming from. The pharmaceuticals that you are then given may suppress the initial symptom for a time, which allows the cinders of an underlying illness to smoulder softly, softly until wildfire breaks out.

Conventional medicine is viewing the body parts as distinct entities. Nothing is connected, which is crazy because, if you think about it, everything in the body is connected, everything is interrelated. Conventional medicine dodges around in the mist and does not take into account (as does restorative medicine) that 'A' might not actually be coming from 'A' but in fact may actually be coming from 'B' or even 'C', and if we were to regulate these ('regulate' being the operative word here), then more than likely 'A' would right itself and neither 'B' nor 'C' would erupt at a later date. By following the conventional form of medicine (drug-based), we are only suppressing the symptom, covering up the underlying cause that is screaming at us to be corrected, yet it is not being corrected because we are not getting to the root cause. When the body talks, it talks for a reason and we ourselves, before anyone else, need to listen to our symptom(s) and learn where they are coming from.

I ask you, just from reading the information above, which would you choose: a medicine that prevents, heals and corrects, or a medicine that suppresses, does not get to the root cause, does not resolve and is just a temporary solution until some other ailment comes along that is connected to the previously suppressed symptom, which will certainly develop into some kind of chronic disease? I can only say that I am tired and I know that, generally, people have grown weary of the medical establishment's methods of not focusing on us as patients, instead offering drugs and diagnostic testing that do not resolve the problem, do not dig deeper, and do not get to the root cause. There is an alternative, and one that works.

All restorative doctors are fully licenced and accredited doctors who come from conventional medicine. They have seen the light and changed their ways, for the better.

Another Way of Looking at Conventional Medicine

Although there are many problem areas with conventional medicine, it is important to understand that restorative medicine is not opposed to it. Conventional medicine has its place, and we certainly wouldn't be where we are today without it. To say it has no place would be sheer stupidity. Surgery and anaesthetics, blood transfusions, penicillin and other antibiotics have changed the world forever; these drugs have expanded the human lifespan greatly over the decades but, unfortunately, not always the quality of it.

Unfortunately, in this ever-changing world there is an abuse of pharmaceutical drugs and an overriding will to make money, whatever the consequence. Consequences and side effects that we are unaware of. Most of the time these drugs cause major health problems in the long run because, as Dr Dzugan explained to me, they are foreign to the body, they are intruders. To use his exact words, "They set up new reactions that declare war on everything they touch." More often than not lifetime drugs cause problems and side effects in another part of the body, which then need to be corrected by another drug, and so it goes on and we get weaker and weaker and then sicker and sicker. Remember: drugs do not heal, they only abate!

By reading this book, and the information in it, you will learn in which direction to go. If you yourself don't know your stuff, how can you ask your doctor and be sure of yourself? How can we make demands or tell them that we want what we want? More often than not, these doctors are set in their ways (no offence meant, it is normal) and are not interested in moving forward. We are just another patient to them. We are the ones that need to push them forward, to introduce them to this amazing medicine, to tweak their curiosity. Unfortunately, the world today is dominated by the pharmaceutical industries and as a consequence, your conventional doctor has never been educated about the health benefits of hormone restorative therapy, nor does he or she understand the quality of life we reap when we embrace this medicine. In a way, we too have been brainwashed by the pharmaceutical establishments into thinking there is a drug for everything, which there is, but with consequences. We are the only ones that can take care of ourselves and protect ourselves; no one else will, so it is up to us to be informed and start loving ourselves. To start researching and start understanding. We are on our own, each and every one of us.

This book offers you the possibility of a better quality of life, a cutting-edge, new age medicine that we all deserve and we all need to know about. As I have already said, every day I hear someone either saying, "My knees are aching", "My bones are breaking", "My heart is not working", "My cholesterol is high", "Those senior moments are getting worse – my brain has completely gone." Their answer? "Oh, it must be my age." Yes, actually that's right, it is their age. It's their body talking to them, telling them something is wrong that needs to be corrected. This is a dysfunctional body. This is the breakdown of optimal body function. This is the body on a spiral descent; going haywire if you like. These are things called 'acquired physiological errors'! The body is dizzy, bobbing around trying to regain its balance, but without restorative intervention you will not regain your balance.

Can we correct this before the volcano erupts, before disease becomes chronic? Can we stop it in its tracks? Yes, yes, and yes! Can you imagine anything better than having the bones of a thirty-year-old, the heart of a thirty-five-year-old and the brains of that wonderful, youthful twenty-five-year-old, and my energy? I am fifty-four but have the energy of a twenty-five-year-old thanks to bioidentical hormone restorative therapy. Oh, and I almost forgot, sex is great again – no kidding, I have gone back in time! We do not have to accept becoming frail, weak and ill in our old age anymore. We believed that this was the only option knocking on our door: a sad, uncomfortable old age. It was something we didn't enjoy, but we accepted it. Well, I can tell you something: we were definitely mistaken! We do not have to follow the present template of growing old, and usual 'run-of-the-mill things' like ending up in a nursing home (which isn't so run-of-the-mill, really – it's terrifying, for me anyway) or becoming a burden on our family. We now have a new template for change.

To me health is everything, there is certainly no quality of life without it but, as I came to realise, health is not just about disease. Health is about feeling good, which was something I had lost; about being full of energy, feeling positive and well, without aches, pains, sadness, depression and weakness. The definition of health is the energy and vitality that I have (thank God for hormone restorative medicine). Health is positive energy, happiness, how we choose to express ourselves, confidence, creative thinking, sexuality. Sexuality is a sixth sense, we are born with it, it is part of us; it is about being radiant, attractive, glowing, confident. There is no beauty without health. With a dysfunctional body we cannot offer all these things to the world and live life to the full. Beauty and old age are in the eye of the beholder, and health is our beholder.

3. HORMONES:
THE DRIVING FORCE OF LIFE

The Common Denominator Factor

Of course, I can see clearly what is running through your mind. You are now saying to yourself, "This woman is claiming that restorative medicine has a cure for everything, from heart disease, depression, weight gain and osteoporosis to migraine, constipation, skin rashes, muscle spasms, insomnia and even sexuality, if you like. Yeah, get that one! There is no way that all these diseases and ailments live under the same roof, I mean there is a doctor for each disease or ailment, right? So that means they are all coming from different places." That is what you are thinking, isn't it? Well, actually, the cause is one. Most symptoms are the body's way of trying to regain homeostasis and balance; it's your body's defence mechanism. Disease should not be treated by suppressing this defence mechanism, but rather by making peace with these systems. There is a common denominator that can make an alliance with all these systems. Talking to Dr Dzugan is an incredible learning experience and he explains things in such a logical manner. It makes sense, kind of what is called 'common sense', really. Something conventional medicine seems to have lost along the way.

It is well known, at least among researchers and qualified restorative doctors, that one of the factors of ageing is due to the naturally occurring decline of hormones, although our lifestyle, incorrect eating habits, toxins, stress levels and environmental factors all contribute to the ageing process. Ageing is multifactorial. You cannot expect to be healthy if you only sleep four or five hours a night, in fact we are at a higher risk of heart attack if we sleep less than seven hours a night. You cannot expect to be well if you don't eat well and sit all day in front of your computer at work, then go home at night to slump into that comfortable armchair in front of the television and devour the biggest plate of pasta or double cheeseburger you can find, together with a huge side plate of French fries and five beers. But I expect you all know that already, even if some of you still do it. You are looking to have a heart attack, right, or perhaps even get Type II diabetes or cancer? Unfortunately, sitting is a new way of life; when I first came to Italy nearly twenty-seven years ago people were always on the move, out in the *campo* (fields) working the land or preparing the beaches for the influx of tourism to come. Yes, we still work the land but more and more people are less willing to do this and want to stay attached to computers and, let's say, a more comfortable life. That's okay, but we need to move as well, we need to get up from our chair and walk around the room, do some push-ups – the more you move, the better. We do not have to go to the gym for hours on end, that only stresses our body, but we do need to move. We are getting more like America every day, which is one of the sickest countries in the western world. Do we really want to follow this way of life?

All the aforementioned are 'fast-forward ageing factors' and are in some way environmental, so can be avoided or managed. Truthfully speaking though, the world we live in today is saturated with environmental hazards from pesticides and preservatives in our food. Foods that contain pesticides, organophosphates and other farming chemicals wreak havoc with our delicate endocrine system and confuse the hormonal conversation within. I will discuss the endocrine system in more detail further on. Pesticides and co. also congest our liver and act like oestrogens, often known as xenoestrogens. We do not want or need these chemical mimicking oestrogens in our body; we do not want to get cancer. We need balance. Other environmental hazards include the damaged and overworked soil that our food is grown in, the water we drink and the air we breathe, although the latter is certainly something we cannot control. But deciding how and what we eat, like organic food, real food, and drinking pure water, are things we can control. Not smoking, getting enough sleep, controlling stress levels and taking up exercise are also things we can control. If we follow the rules, these things can help us avoid certain diseases such as obesity, diabetes (just because we have a genetic predisposition does not necessarily mean the switch will be activated; we need to follow the rules), hypertension, coronary heart disease and cancer.

But let's get back to the part about the naturally occurring decline in hormone levels. This is 'The Major Ager', this is the real culprit, the detonator to age-related diseases! This was something we definitely could not avoid or prevent until now, and which brings with it a change in physiology, or a breakdown in physiological function. Declining hormone levels are almost always associated with chronic illness and all age-related diseases. This is what I call the common denominator to ageing: hormonal loss. Dr Dzugan believes that, by correcting physiology and therefore restoring the body to optimal levels with the use of bioidentical hormones, vitamins, supplements and minerals, which are all interrelated, we can slow the ageing process and use restorative medicine to treat age-related diseases.

Conventional medicine does not get this. They want us to fill up our medicine cabinets with pharmaceutical, chemical drugs and hang onto dear life *Every Which Way but Loose*, or a sequel to it, *Any Which Way You Can*. What quality of life is there if you are stuck in a wheelchair, can't think straight, co-ordinate or remember anything because of a severe degradation of hormones? What quality of life is there if we are frightened to move in case a bone snaps and disintegrates into powder? What quality of life is there if we are just sitting there waiting for our heart to give in, or for cancer to explode? We need to understand our hormones, or rather the decline of them, and how they interact with each other and other bodily systems that determine how we age. This is the common denominator.

Bioidentical hormones are the true strength to restorative medicine and are vital to getting you back on track. An imbalance of hormones fast-forwards the ageing process. With imbalanced hormones you cannot truly be well. With controlled hormones at optimal levels we regain our balance, our love of life and our sleep – wonderful sleep. Remember the days when you slept so well and woke up not feeling tired? Good sleep is one of the cornerstones of health. Without balanced hormones sleep is impossible and without sleep hormones will never be balanced, it is a vicious circle. Without sleep we cannot regenerate our health. Without sleep optimal health will remain elusive. Sleep is an 'age saver' and is imperative to health. Hormones are more powerful than drugs and, I say it again, they are the essence of life itself. Hormones regulate every bodily function: sleep, growth, blood pressure, heartbeat, breathing – without them we would simply die. They control muscle tone, build bone, make us fat or thin, maintain correct levels of sugar in the blood and tissue, control women's menstrual cycles, make men males, rule the passage of time and the voyage into menopause. Without optimal levels of hormones our body slows down and becomes inefficient, dysfunctional and eventually chronic disease sets in. We, the laypersons, need to recognise the telltale signs of hormonal decline. Memory loss – where did I park my car? What's his name, my best friend? Sleepless nights – always tired. Depressed and anxious. Weight gain, breathlessness, high blood pressure, high cholesterol levels, and every other day you hear someone has got cancer. Things that we didn't have when we were young. It's when a hormonal imbalance occurs that disease can step in. Miscommunication prevails and mistakes are made. The fact is, we begin our descent into ageing and its related illnesses because our hormones decline, not the other way round. In other words, our hormones do not decline because we age or become ill, we become ill because our hormones decline. When you restore them, you will protect yourself.

As I said before, my life was definitely on a downhill path, both mentally and physically, until I restored my body. In my case, hormonal loss played a great part in mental and emotional symptoms. I am ashamed to admit this, but there were times when my body had decided to turn against me, in the perimenopause phase, when I would scream like a mad woman, throw myself in a corner, huddle down and cry, and for no good reason. Life had just become too much for me. I lost the will to go out and enjoy myself, I lost confidence, I did not like socialising anymore; something I used to love doing. I didn't enjoy getting dressed up anymore – in Italy everyone gets dressed up. It's a fantastic country for fashion. I should know, I used to design my own clothes, from silk shirts to leather jackets. Fashion was my first love, but restorative medicine has now taken its place. I made the decision to reinstate my health, my vitality and my emotional state – had I not, divorce was on the cards. Once you realise the immense benefits and joys that bioidentical hormones can bring you, you will understand life again and see how wonderful it can be. Without balanced hormones, your life and body will only decline, slowly but surely! Why do that to yourself?

You are reading this book and I am so glad you have joined me on this wonderful journey, and would be thrilled if you choose to take control of your life. Taking control of your hormones means being in charge of your life. By restoring my body I took charge of my life and I am so glad I did; I see and feel the results every day. It can change your life for the better too, and save you from pain, discomfort and disease.

Without a doubt you will meet people along the way who will try and tell you that you are foolish or reckless – I certainly did. The usual statement is, "Hormones are dangerous, you must be mad mixing in that stuff!" These are people who unfortunately do not understand but I chose not judge them for it; I rather pitied them for it. When they tried to criticise me, I told them that they didn't understand. I told them I was not experimenting or risking my life; that I was, in actual fact, saving it. Join me on this journey. You are still holding this book in your hands, so know exactly where you want to go. You are not self-involved, vanity-obsessed or mad – you are you and you want to be you. With the precision, power and expertise of restorative medicine you will be the 'you' you once were! Mentally, physically and emotionally – a rolling stone.

The second half of your life can be something to look forward to instead of dread. You have the worldly experience of a mature person and at the same time you can have the health, vitality and energy of someone half your age. This new medicine is your greatest defence against cancer, heart attacks and Alzheimer's. Your brain, your precious brain – you can have a perfectly working brain, no more foggy thinking. I even got my sense of humour back.

So, let's move onto the complicated part. This book will help you to build a better life, I promise. Read through it one step at a time and you will get to your final destination and reach your goal. To live life to the full for a long time.

Hormones! What Are They?

The foundation of the endocrine system are the hormones and glands. Everyone's hormones are as unique as their fingerprint and their DNA, or as that beautiful white snowflake we see falling in the winter.

The hormonal system, which is commonly known as the endocrine system, controls many important physiological functions. Most of the body's hormones are produced by the glands of the endocrine system. These glands include the hypothalamus, pituitary gland, pineal, thyroid and parathyroids, adrenal glands, pancreas, ovaries and testes. Knowing exactly what a hormone is and how these hormones work within the endocrine network is an important place to start if you want to understand the complexities of the human body!

Hormones decline with age and already become slowly evident at the age of thirty, shifting into second gear at forty, then into third at fifty, and accelerating into fourth and fifth as time goes on. Hormones decline because the endocrine glands cannot keep up the same production of hormones we made in our younger years. As Dr Dzugan defines it, "Age is natural hormonal castration."

In the beginning, there is only a slight deterioration and few complaints, which you may think are unimportant, but these are the first signs of a shift in your hormones. Maybe you're not sleeping right, or your energy levels have dropped slightly. Maybe you are more irritable than normal, your periods may have become a little erratic, and your breasts may be painful, swollen and lumpy. These are the same signs experienced by many old women you see every day on the street, or in nursing homes or care centres. These women were once like you. These are the women who now have Alzheimer's, have had cancer, strokes, heart attacks, and have osteoporosis. The difference is, they didn't have the option of restorative medicine and bioidentical hormones to turn to. We do. Think about it: we do not need to become ill like them.

You may, like I did, hear your friends complain about endometriosis; sudden weight gain, especially around the middle, becoming thicker rather than fatter, changing shape, mixed-up thinking and feelings, uterine fibroids and migraines. Cold hands and/or feet may happen; that was one of mine, I was always cold, especially my hands and feet. These are telltale signs, warning signs. Towards the end there is total devastation in the body; that is why people in their eighties look so old – their movements, their brain, their skin, their bent-up weak bodies are showing us they are old: the machine is no longer functioning at optimal levels.

Because there is a gradual decline, most people don't even realise it is happening. The usual thought is, "It's just my age." We keep saying 'age', it's all to do with age, which of course it is, but there are two types of ageing: biological and chronological. We are all going to age, without doubt, but we can choose how we age. What restorative doctors say is, "We are only as healthy as our weakest hormone." Take this ageing process into your own hands and look towards restorative medicine, build your body back up, restore your body, which ultimately slows down the ageing process and, in some cases, reverses it. You need to recognise these first niggling complaints before they get a hold; your body is talking to you. This is one of the reasons I am writing this book, to help you understand and make you aware.

Life Set Into Motion

Hormones affect every bodily process and have an enormous influence on the way we look and the way we feel. They are vital for repair and are the most powerful agent in the regulation of an optimal physiology. They are vital parts of the neuro-endocrine-immune system. Hormones transport information from the brain to the glands, then from the glands to the cells, and from the cells to the brain. When there is a hormonal imbalance, havoc erupts within the endocrine system and trouble begins. Basically, when the endocrine system goes into default, it creates problems with other bodily systems, including the immune, cardiovascular and gastrointestinal systems.

A hormone is a chemical substance produced or secreted by a gland. Hormones are the body's chemical messengers that send instructions or information from one set of cells to another. No less than sixty-trillion cells are affected to a certain degree by these extraordinary hormones; imagine the horror upon horrors when there is a decline and the talking between these cells and hormones becomes incoherent. Looking at it logically, as we are made up of cells, it seems a good idea to try and keep these agents (hormones) in our body and at optimal levels. What do you think? From the moment the umbilical cord is cut and our first breath is taken, hormones are key to how we function, grow and age. Optimal levels of hormones signify health, quality of life and longevity, full stop.

As I mentioned previously, the endocrine system is made up of various glands. These glands release important hormones, such as pregnenolone, oestrogens, testosterone, progesterone, DHEA, cortisol, aldosterone, melatonin and thyroid hormones (which are of major interest to restorative medicine) directly into the bloodstream, which then search out cells fitted with special receptors. The release of these hormones is controlled by a master gland in the brain called the hypothalamus. Their goal is to reach their specific destination; each specific hormone is designed to deliver specific information to a specific cell group or organ throughout the body. Once the hormone has been recognised, metabolised and used, it then travels to the liver to be broken down and expelled from the body. If just one part of this process fails, a hormonal imbalance can occur.

HPA-Axis Diagram

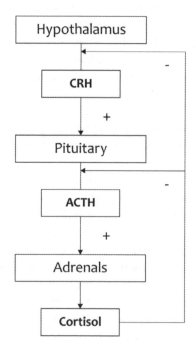

Hormonal decline is no joke, as I found out. When there is a hormonal decline, it can cause a negative impact on the production and levels of other hormones. When even one hormone is in decline, the imbalance will be closely followed by the rest, which will cause a downward cascade of all bodily functions. Hormones talk to each other; they are all interrelated, mutually pumping each other up or slowing each other down to achieve the correct balance. They are players of a team that is responsible for maintaining our health. The definition of imbalanced hormones is disease and health problems. Declining hormones set the wheels in motion – the word 'hormone' comes from the Greek language and means 'to set in motion'; very appropriate.

The once well-oiled machine then bumps along sending messages to other organs to release incorrect levels of other hormones, which in turn cause other organs to release incorrect levels of another hormone. This is turn will cause a hormonal imbalance and provoke the body to become dysfunctional and age. When the endocrine network is 100% and working fluidly, we will feel great, look great and will be able to hold off nearly all infections and chronic disease. A healthy endocrine system is upmost to a happy and healthy you and, at the end of the day, is one of the factors that determine our biological age.

Teamwork

The hypothalamus is the gland that is roughly the size of an almond and is located in the lower central part of the brain. It plays a role in growth, appetite, conversion of food into energy (metabolism), blood pressure, your level of sexual activity, your mood and your responses to heat and cold. It is the major link between the endocrine system and nervous system. These two systems are the most profoundly affected by regulation. Regulation means that the organs and tissues are able to respond appropriately to a stimulus; they understand, the message is received loud and clear. Each system has a feedback on the other and works in harmony when functioning at optimum. The nervous system works at breakneck speeds, regulating within seconds; the endocrine system, on the other hand, functions more slowly and its adjustments can take from minutes to hours to develop.

The hypothalamus is often called the hormone receptionist or call centre, and not without reason as it receives messages that come from the brain, which in turn release hormonal messages to the pituitary gland, which is located just below the hypothalamus and is attached by nerve fibres. It is the keeper of internal balance and homeostasis, and acts as the call centre for most of the body's hormonal systems.

Pituitary Gland

The pituitary gland is about the size of a pea and located at the base of the brain. It produces hormones that control several endocrine glands, and is divided into two distinct parts: the anterior and posterior lobes, each one producing specific hormones when prompted by the hypothalamus.

Pituitary Gland

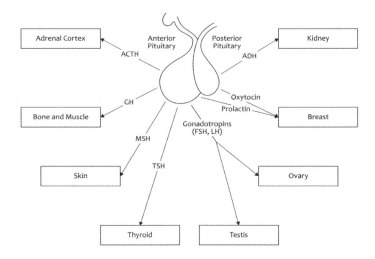

Hormones produced by the pituitary gland are released into the bloodstream, as with all endocrine hormones, and stimulate target glands, such as the thyroid, adrenal and reproductive glands, to secrete their hormones. The target glands respond to the specific hormone because it bears receptors for that specific hormone. In other words, receptors bind to the given cell membrane or organ (which is genetically programmed) like a key in a lock or, as I like to say, like a puzzle piece that fits securely into place, producing the requested effect on the metabolism and function of the target organ.

Pineal Gland

The pineal gland is a pine-shaped gland, hence its name. It was the last gland of the endocrine system to be discovered and is located deep in the brain, where it is lodged in a tiny cave behind the ocular nerves, and is about the size of a raisin. It works closely with the hypothalamus to help govern various biological rhythms, it is our body's timekeeper and it knows our age. The pineal gland is photosensitive, meaning it is activated by light. The retinas of the eyes send information, or communicate, through the sympathetic nerve system (I will talk about this later) to the pineal gland, which then translates these impulses to release certain hormones in the brain – there is a lot of talking going on. The pineal gland's primary function is to produce and secrete the hormone melatonin. Melatonin is the hormone that is associated with the sleep-wake circadian (daily) cycle.

Autonomic Nervous System

If you remember, I spoke earlier about the link between the endocrine system and nervous system. The autonomic nervous system (ANS) is part of the central nervous system, which is composed of the brain and spinal cord, and regulates (talks to or instructs) organs in our body such as the heart, intestines, stomach and bladder. The ANS works to control the muscles of these organs, as well as the muscles in the eye, skin and blood vessels. It also works with the endocrine system, mainly through the hypothalamus, to control the secretion of hormones. The hypothalamus is always busy.

The Sympathetic and Parasympathetic Nervous Systems – the Migraine Enigma

Every system in the body has to be working at optimum for us to be truly well. The ANS is made up of three parts. The sympathetic nervous system and the parasympathetic nervous system are what I would like to talk about for the moment. I mentioned in Chapter 1 that Dr Dzugan developed an effective method of treatment for migraine. More than 85% of his patients got complete relief from migraine pain and related symptoms following this individualised approach. In other words, 85% of patients got rock-solid relief! Even patients who had difficult-to-treat migraines, and who had had them for more than thirty years, got relief. Absolutely no drugs involved.

The balance between both of these systems is critical for the prevention of migraine and other medical disorders. To achieve balance between the two nervous systems, Dr Dzugan initially balances four other systems, which simultaneously go on to balance the sympathetic and parasympathetic nervous systems. The four systems are:

The neurohormonal system (which I discuss later).
Here Dr Dzugan's goal is to restore hormones to levels that are appropriate for the individual, so as to regain balance.

The pineal gland.
Here the goal is to reset the function of this gland. The pineal gland balances the cyclic production of the hormone melatonin and also the neurotransmitter serotonin. Serotonin is the precursor of melatonin (I discuss neurotransmitters

in more detail later). Both melatonin and serotonin are key players in migraine. If we reset the pineal gland we regain balance. Balance is a big word in restorative medicine.

The digestive system.
Restoring balance within the digestive system is a critical part of the migraine cure.

Last, but certainly not least, Dr Dzugan's approach includes the balance of magnesium ions. To obtain harmony there has to be balance between two critical minerals – magnesium and calcium. An imbalance in the ratio of these two substances is a crucial factor in migraine.

Migraine is a result of an imbalance among several critical systems in the body. When there is a culmination of imbalances they are reflected in the sympathetic and parasympathetic nervous systems. So, when balance is achieved between all the other systems, harmony is restored within these two complimentary nervous systems. When there is an imbalance within these two nervous systems our pain threshold is reduced in the brain's nociceptive system. Nociceptive pain happens when nerve endings, which are called nociceptors, are irritated. The nociceptive system controls this pain. Pain can be mild, severe, acute or chronic.

Both the sympathetic and parasympathetic nervous systems work continuously and simultaneously, but at varying degrees. Nearly every organ in the body has a double set of nerves which are provided by the ANS – one is the sympathetic and the other is the parasympathetic. What this means is that both systems are continually having an impact on the same organ, but their impact differs both in degree and effect. There is a kind of balancing act between the two: the sympathetic nervous system is an energy-giver and is known as the 'fight or flight' system, whereas the parasympathetic system is a calming system which brings the body back into equilibrium or homeostasis. Balance is everything.

To give you an example how it works, the sympathetic system controls the body's response to emergencies such as a tiger running at you to attack you – your heart rate goes up, the adrenaline in your bloodstream is greatly increased, giving you amazing strength (you are getting ready to fight that tiger off – "Oh boy, it ain't getting its teeth into me!"), blood pressure goes up, breathing rate increases, digestion slows or stops, your pupils dilate and you begin to sweat. When the tiger turns away and decides you are not good enough to eat, the parasympathetic nervous system takes over – the body calms; phew, you wipe the sweat off your forehead. The heart rate slowly returns to normal, adrenaline decreases and your temporary strength dissipates, blood pressure decreases, breathing rate slows, digestion resumes, pupils contract and sweating ceases. Back to normal.

Of course, you are not going to have a tiger running at you every day so your stressors won't be as dramatic as that – that was just to give you an example of how things work. We always have some kind of stressors in our lives: emotional stress, stress from poor dietary habits and so on. The sympathetic and parasympathetic systems are continually at work, one dominating the other, trying to maintain balance. The stressors I mentioned previously can cause an imbalance between the two nervous systems, mainly because these stressors create an imbalance within our other bodily systems. When there is an imbalance within the other bodily systems our sympathetic and parasympathetic nervous systems are fighting for their lives. They cannot find homeostasis because there is continual upset in our body. If we adjust or reset the other systems then bingo – your migraines will be gone forever. You can now have peace at last.

Adrenal Glands

The adrenal glands are two orange, triangular glands that sit on the top of each kidney near the spine, just underneath the last rib. Males' adrenals are usually slightly heavier than females'.

The adrenal glands are strategically placed near the aorta, the major artery of the body, and the major vein, called the vena cava. This allows for a very rapid response to hormonal messages relayed through the bloodstream. Isn't the body incredible? I am touched by wonder and pleasure every time I learn about the wisdom of our own body. Also, the adrenals are placed in close proximity to the liver, pancreas, major fat-storage areas and the kidneys. Once again, our bodily wisdom has placed them there for a reason. These organs require rapid and immediate communication with the adrenal hormones.

The adrenals are about three inches in length and are made up of a medulla (inner part) and a cortex (outer part). The cortex consists of three zones:

Adrenal Gland

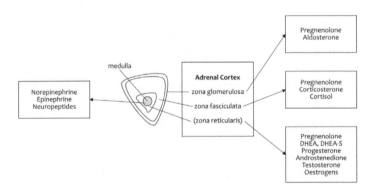

The zona glomerulosa, which produces aldosterone and pregnenolone. This helps to maintain blood volume and pressure by way of controlling the blood balance of sodium to potassium.

The zona fasciculata, which produces cortisol, the stress hormone and pregnenolone. (We will cover this later).

The zona reticularis, which produces pregnenolone, progesterone, DHEA and DHEA-S, and a small amount of oestrogens and testosterone. Mainly though, the latter two hormones are produced by the ovaries and testes. After menopause, all our sex hormones are made by the adrenal glands.

There is a special relationship between cortisol and DHEA (DHEA is the precursor to oestrogens and testosterone). The cortisol-to-DHEA ratio decreases when we are calm, but increases when we are ill or under acute stress. Not only are optimal hormonal levels extremely important in restorative medicine, so are the ratios between them.

The medulla produces adrenaline (epinephrine), which is secreted from the hypothalamus in response to the 'tiger attack'. This is the sympathetic nervous system response, the 'fight or flight' reaction.

Each of the three zones in the adrenal cortex contains cholesterol, which is converted into the hormone pregnenolone. Adrenocorticotropic hormone (ACTH) plays a significant role in the production of cholesterol. Let me explain. One of the main releasing-hormone messengers from the hypothalamus is corticotropin-releasing hormone (CRH), also known as corticotropin-releasing factor (CRF). The release of this hormone tells the pituitary gland to produce a specific quantity of ACTH. Because of this mechanism, the body determines how much cortisol it requires. Cortisol is known as the stress hormone. I will talk more about cortisol later.

So ACTH is secreted in response to the needs of the body under normal and stressed conditions, via the pituitary gland, where it travels through the bloodstream to the adrenal cortex. It then binds to the walls of the adrenal cells, which initiate a chain reaction of intracellular enzymes that release cholesterol within the cells. Cholesterol is then used inside the adrenal cells to manufacture pregnenolone. No matter which adrenal hormone is being produced, pregnenolone is always the first and foremost hormone in the cascade.

Pregnenolone goes on to make a cascade of other steroid hormones, including progesterone, DHEA, testosterone, oestrogens and cortisol.

The adrenals' hormones are prompted by the hypothalamus and go on to communicate with the pituitary. The pituitary then communicates with the thyroid and back to the adrenals – there is a lot of talking going on here. Because of this so-called loop, the adrenals talk to all the other hormones and guide them; they (the adrenals) direct the rest of the endocrine system to keep all the hormones balanced. The adrenals are very important, in fact critical, in the make-up or breakdown of our health. They are the 'leaders of the pack'; the song will continue to play at its best when the adrenals are working at optimum. Optimal functioning of the adrenal glands is vital for hormone production; a direct result of adrenal insufficiency is a hormonal imbalance.

The Neurohormonal System and the HPA Axis: Hypothalamus, Pituitary and Adrenals

The neurohormonal system is a network of hormones, hormone messages, hormone receptors and nerve pathways which work together to maintain balance among the various systems in our body. These are all key factors to restorative medicine and its programme. A major component of the neurohormonal system is the hypothalamic/pituitary/adrenal axis (all of which we have spoken about above), or the HPA axis, and how they are all interconnected.

The HPA axis is key to achieving homeostasis; each component works in concert and is affected by environment and lifestyle. If we have been out of sync, such as a hormonal imbalance, not sleeping, suffering from poor diet and stress, the HPA axis will be off balance. To achieve harmony within the body, all elements must be balanced. Restorative medicine looks to reset the HPA axis, helping us to live a long, headache-free, peaceful life.

4. BIOIDENTICAL VERSUS SYNTHETIC HORMONES

There is a big difference between bioidentical and synthetic hormones, and how they work within our bodies. Something like good and bad, black and white, devil or saint. It's as simple as that.

Bioidentical Hormones

Bioidentical hormones are not pharmaceutical drugs. They are biologically identical to the hormones that are produced in our body, identical in molecular structure – hormone replicas. They come from soya, wild yam and other plant extracts that are bioengineered in a lab to become an exact copy of the human hormone. A good example is man-made progesterone that is synthesised in a laboratory from the molecule of so-called diosgenin, found in wild yam – the result is molecularly identical. Wild yam does not contain progesterone so, to achieve a natural progesterone result, it has to be made in the laboratory. This ensures that the progesterone is 100% bioidentical or natural to the requirements of the human body.

Nature works perfectly with our body, in harmony. Being exactly the same in terms of molecular structure, our bodies know exactly how to take these natural substances and metabolise them in precisely the same way they metabolise the body's natural molecules, using them for energy, repair and regeneration, excreting them when necessary and without difficulty.

Because of their nature, natural, bioidentical hormones are non-patentable, therefore uninteresting to the pharmaceutical companies because of low profit margins – this is one of the reasons why we hear so little about them. No money to be made! Fight the big fight.

Synthetic Hormones

Synthetic hormones are completely different from bioidentical hormones – black and white. A synthetic hormone is a substance that is not found in nature, rather, it is reinvented from nature so as to be patented. You may say, "So what! What's the big deal?" But the deal is real, and big. The deal, for instance, can lead to death by heart attack or breast cancer. The devil or a saint. You make the choices.

"So what!" you say. Let me give you an insight: chemically altering – adding or subtracting one or two atoms of a molecule – makes a big difference in how the body is affected and even very small amounts can create major effects. For example, the difference between testosterone and oestradiol (a type of oestrogen) is only one hydrogen atom and a couple of double bonds. Now just imagine what pharmaceutical companies do to perfectly natural hormones when they add whole chains of molecules, and what effects these have on our bodies. They are not making a drug that works better, but by doing this they are inventing one that behaves similarly yet differently enough to be patentable, and one that does us more damage in the long run.

Unlike natural or bioidentical hormones, synthetic, alien or pseudohormones cannot be metabolised safely and efficiently without producing toxic by-products. The fact is that the body has an inbuilt system that metabolises bioidentical hormones easily. For every natural hormone there are enzymes and other chemicals that work exclusively to produce a smooth, non-problematic, side-effect-free landing. For centuries upon centuries, or forever, let's say, our experienced bodies have handled natural hormones and have coped very well but, when your patented, chemically-altered, drug-like hormone steps in, the body becomes confused. Basically, the body's biological infrastructure is not set up to accept these alien molecules.

Although both bioidentical and synthetic hormones are created in a laboratory atmosphere, this does not mean – again, I stress this – that they are one and the same. Synthetic hormones are foreign compounds that are never actually produced inside the body. Bioidentical hormones are natural to the human body and provide many health benefits.

Let's Talk This Over: DES

I just want to go back in time for a second, so you can have a better understanding about synthetic hormones and how nasty they are. DES (diethylstilbestrol) was the first synthetic hormone. If you remember, I mentioned DES at the beginning of the book. My mother took it when she was pregnant with my sister – and look what happened to my sister. DES was invented in 1938 and came onto the marketplace round about 1941, and millions of women were given this ugly drug. It was banned in 1975 when it was proven to cause cervical cancer. It has since been found to have even more profound side effects, spanning to the next generation to those who had been exposed to it *in utero* (in the womb).

DES was largely prescribed to prevent miscarriages and other pregnancy complications. My mother had a dermoid cyst removed along with her left ovary when she was twenty-two-weeks pregnant and was subsequently given three shots (injections) of DES. My sister, who was exposed to DES *in utero*, got bilateral breast cancer, had infertility problems, had multiple miscarriages and her only son was born prematurely – these are typical side effects of this nasty drug. She also had a hysterectomy, but that could have been due to the tamoxifen she was instructed to take due to her breast cancers. She had her hysterectomy in between both cancers.

Tamoxifen works differently on the uterus than on the breast. Tamoxifen (Nolvadex®) is given to help prevent or inhibit cancer growth in oestrogen-sensitive tumours in the breast, but unfortunately, has various adverse side effects, one of which is that it stimulates hyperplasia and endometrial cancer. Tamoxifen and raloxifene (Evista®) are marketed as SERMs (selective oestrogen receptor modulators). SERMs are selective, as the name suggests, so they only block oestrogen from one type of cell: the breast tissue cell. However, our body has many, many oestrogen receptor sites throughout, all of which are structured slightly differently, depending on what cell they are in. Unfortunately, SERMS can activate oestrogen's actions in other cells. So, here's the deal: tamoxifen inhibits in the breast but stimulates in the uterus. Women who take tamoxifen (Nolvadex), like my sister, to protect against breast cancer, actually increase their risk of uterine cancer. It can double or triple the risk of uterine cancer, and it also increases the risk of blood clots. Other side effects in oestrogen(s)-sensitive tissues range from urinary incontinence, worsening of hot flushes and other menopausal discomfort, leg cramps and stroke to blood clots in legs and lungs.

Raloxifene has selective oestrogen activity for bone, meaning it helps maintain bone structure. So the only thing you may get out of it is that it may help prevent osteoporosis, but it can potentially increase the risk of stress fractures after five years of taking it.

HRT Today

OK, so here's the deal today with HRT. The drug, Premarin® – do you know the full story? Premarin is a horse oestrogen. It is derived from the pee of pregnant mares. Some people may, mistakenly, believe that, because of this, it can be classed as being natural and is safe. This is not the case. Although Premarin does contain oestrogens natural to humans (e.g. oestrone), it also contains oestrogens natural to a horse (equilin, equilenin). What is our body going to do with these horse oestrogens? We are not horses. Premarin is not bioidentical to human requirements. Our body cannot read horse hormones and certainly cannot talk to them.

Premarin® (oestrogen replacement therapy) came onto the market in the same year it was approved by the FDA in 1942, but has only been widely marketed since the 1960s, and was designed to help menopausal symptoms. This horse-oestrogen hormone was then found to cause cancer of the uterus (endometrial cancer). Between 1970 and 1975 it was estimated that fifteen thousand women contracted endometrial cancer – that is a five-year period; incredible. It was a real epidemic.

Even after this epidemic increase in uterine cancer became apparent, instead of pulling it from their shelves, the pharmaceutical company decided to make another drug. They took the natural progesterone, converted it into progestin, chemically altering it so it could be patented along with its life-threatening side effects, and called it Provera®. These two drugs, Provera and Premarin, were then put together to prevent the equine oestrogen causing uterine cancer and to increase the market share to women with uteruses. Thus, Prempro® was born – Prem from Premarin and Pro from Provera®. A pill that fits all – all types of women, a static dose, not rhythmic, as would happen in a woman's natural cycle, and not individually tailored. So now there was a drug that not only contained one alien hormone, but two: horse oestrogen and progestin. This was supposedly meant to make things better. Unfortunately this was not the case. Again, there were problems. This combo drug proved fatal; the addition of progestin made matters even worse. Various studies showed there to be an increase in breast cancer and heart disease.

In 1997 a major study called the Women's Health Initiative (WHI) began. This clinical trial consisted of 161,000 healthy menopausal women from ages fifty to seventy-nine, and was spread over forty different clinics in America and looked at both these chemical hormones – horse oestrogen and progestin. The study was set up to demonstrate that long-term treatment with Premarin plus Provera reduced the risk of osteoporosis, colorectal cancer, dementia and heart disease, and at the same time improved overall well-being. Originally, the main purpose of patented HRT was to put a stop to those dreadful hot flushes we have to put up with, one of the most common symptoms of menopause. Most menopausal women find that hot flushes, night sweats, sleeping difficulties and mood swings are transitory and last only as long as it takes the body to adapt to the lower hormone levels. However, more important and permanent changes such as drying and thinning skin and vaginal membranes, foggy memory and decreased urinary tract tone, and later developments such as heart disease, osteoporosis and cognitive problems, all become more apparent with age unless hormones are replaced. Think bioidentical, not synthetic. Synthetic hormones are bad, ugly and nasty products. Bioidentical are good, good, good.

The WHI study was due to last eight and a half years but when it revealed that the risks of HRT outweighed the benefits, the study was suddenly terminated at five and a half years in 2002. The conclusion of this unfinished study was that the use of both Premarin (alien oestrogens) and Provera (alien progesterone/progestin) caused breast cancer and did not produce the supposed benefits such as protection against cardiovascular disease, strokes or cognitive loss. Nor did it improve mood or sexual dissatisfaction, although it did help hot flushes and night sweats. However, the big surprise that came out of this study was not the breast cancer risk – this had always been on the cards, albeit it had been downplayed by the supposed protection or benefits of this drug. After only four years of taking Prempro®, women showed a 26% increase in invasive breast cancer. And, what was worse, the cancers that occurred in this 26% were slightly larger and more advanced and were more likely to spread to nearby lymph nodes.

So, 'The Big Surprise!'

The most devastating finding of the WHI was that HRT's cardiovascular protection was a myth, one big illusion. Prior to this study, HRT had been associated with a 30% to 50% reduction in coronary problems, but the WHI study showed that Prempro® increased the risk of heart disease by 29% overall and a shocking 81% during the first year of use. Also, the risk of strokes was heightened by 41%, while the risk of blood clots in the lungs and legs was doubled. But, to give Prempro its fair due, a slight reduction in colorectal cancer was shown and fewer hip fractures were associated with it.

Controversy

The aftermath of the WHI study brought with it a lot of negativity. A frenzied media went on to misrepresent bioidentical hormones by not distinguishing between the synthetic form of hormones and bioidentical hormones. The consequences were not good, and controversy set in. It made women wary, apprehensive, leading them into retreat, leaving them to suffer menopausal symptoms unnecessarily. They didn't know where to turn or what to do, and any hormone became a bad word, whether synthetic or bioidentical, whether a birth control pill or HRT. In fact, the birth control pill is a similar drug to HRT and is made out of mutated synthetic oestrogens and fake progesterone. I realise that the contraceptive pill may have been taken for a different reason but basically it contains the same synthetic hormones that are in HRT. Breast cancer risk is increased with the extended use of the patented oestrogen, progestin oral contraceptive pill (usually ethinyl estradiol and progestin), and postmenopausal synthetic oestrogen-progestin regime (HRT). Studies show that five or more years of HRT (not bioidentical hormone replacement therapy) increases the risk of breast cancer by 30% to 40% compared to non-users.

Women taking HRT may suppress hot flushes but they do NOT improve their long-term health, they only exacerbate the situation. The only *safe* way to accomplish an improvement in long-term health is look towards restorative medicine and get in balance.

What we desperately need to understand – and I cannot stress this enough – is that synthetic and bioidenticals are not one and the same. Bioidentical hormones are safe when used correctly. Synthetic hormones are just not. The truth of the matter is, it is when our own hormones decline or go into default that things become dangerous. We rarely see chronic disease in youth, when hormones are balanced. This is the major reason for keeping our hormonal levels optimal with bioidentical hormones and not with synthetic hormones, which disrupt our endocrine system by sending misleading chemical messages, eventually creating a drastic situation.

So Where Do We Go From Here? Optimal Hormone Levels!

We've understood that we need to reach optimal health, at whatever age, if we want to live a long and fun-filled life. To do this, we must obtain optimal hormone levels, each balanced perfectly and with the correct ratios, so as to mimic our healthiest prime.

Optimal hormone levels are the key factor to overall health and longevity. When I say optimal levels I don't mean optimal levels for your age, I mean optimal levels that you had when you were young. Let me explain.

If you were to go to your doctor with your blood or urine tests in your hand, taking into account your age, whatever that might be, and your reference values were normal, he would look at them and tell you how great you were doing for your age. But we don't want that, we don't want the hormone levels that are normal for a person of your age – that would be hormone levels that are in decline. The objective is to bring our hormone levels to a youthful, energetic level; to a level we had when we were twenty-five. We want the correct amount, not too much, nor too little – we want balance. Twenty-five-year-olds are at their hormonal peak; that is why restorative medicine uses these levels as a guide.

To bring your hormones to optimal levels, Dr Dzugan will request a detailed medical history and intricate blood tests that tell him everything he needs to know about your state of health. From this Dr Dzugan can then work on your individualised programme.

5. CHOLESTEROL AND STEROID HORMONES

Cholesterol: the Manufacturing Plant

Cholesterol is a vital substance in our body. We need it to enable the body to function; it builds us up and keeps us strong. Without it we will not go far. Cholesterol is not what you have been brainwashed into thinking it is. It really is very important in keeping us healthy. For the moment, I just want to touch on, or introduce you to, cholesterol, but we will cover it in more detail further along in the book.

Cholesterol has many important functions in the body, including the building of cells, the routine repair of tissue and the creation of hormones. Cells and hormones are pretty important components for keeping us alive or, in the worst-case scenario, dead. For now, I would like to talk about the connection between cholesterol and steroid hormone production. I am not talking about those nasty synthetic steroid hormones that you are probably thinking about right now. The ones that bodybuilders use so they can impair their kidney function or stunt their skeletal growth, or the ones hospitals use to suppress inflammation. I am talking about endogenous steroid hormones – this simply means they are created by and in the body, which is a natural part of normal function.

Cholesterol is vitally important for the production of all steroid hormones; it is the 'site of production'. The first hormone to be manufactured from cholesterol, with help of a specific enzyme, is pregnenolone, which is the precursor to all the other hormones, including the sex hormones.

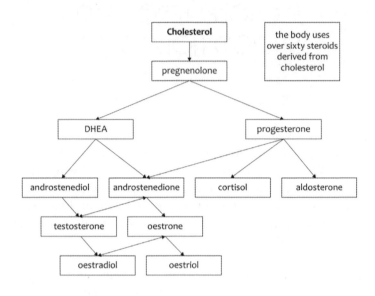

Metabolism of Cholesterol
(simplified version)

The Minor and Major Hormones

Oestrogens, progesterone, testosterone, pregnenolone and DHEA are what are called minor hormones. Oestrogens and progesterone decline drastically in perimenopause – starting to feel the change? Women have testosterone too, although at lower levels than men. Testosterone enhances our sex drive and fantasy levels. It affects sexual sensitivity, nipple sensitivity, clitoris size and sensitivity, and the ability to reach orgasm. There is more information on testosterone later in the book, as it has many more important qualities we need to pay attention to.

Thyroid, insulin, adrenaline and cortisol are all majors. When our minors default and go into decline, our majors increase. This is why we don't feel so good; our balance is out of whack. Sex drive is gone with the wind, sleepless nights are a never-ending story, crazy hot flushes and night sweats torture us, distracted, absent-minded moments leave us bewildered, bloated stomachs ruin that figure-hugging dress you want to wear tonight. With low or imbalanced hormones our body is in a vulnerable state which is potentially dangerous to our health.

The reason I differentiate between major and minor hormones is because we have major and minor hormone systems in our body. The major hormones are essential to life, whereas minor hormones are responsible for fine-tuning and a feeling of well-being. Each hormonal system communicates with the other and needs to be in balance for us to feel well and for our bodies to work at optimum.

Oestrogens

So let's start off with the most famous of sex hormones – oestrogens – and one of the female monitors. We are born with one to two million undeveloped eggs in our ovaries and, by the time we reach puberty and start menstruating, approximately only 300,000 immature egg cells (or follicles) remain. Following this, an average of 600 follicles die per month, which are not replaced. By the time we reach menopause, there are no eggs left and, as eggs are the main producer of female hormones, this is the reason why we slowly become deficient.

Oestrogens are produced in the ovaries and work in harmony with progesterone, another main hormone produced in the ovaries. Oestrogens and progesterone prepare the lining of the uterus for pregnancy; together, they also nurture and maintain the growth and regeneration of our female reproductive tissues.

Some oestrogens such as oestradiol and oestrone are the strongest hormones in the female body; they have approximately three hundred different tissues that are set up or equipped with oestrogen(s) receptors. Literally, our body has oestrogen(s) sites everywhere. What this means is that the oestrogen(s) levels in our body have an enormous influence over a vast range of tissues and organs. Oestrogens have over four hundred crucial functions.

Oestrogens act on the brain, muscles, liver, gut, uterus and urinary tract. Do you often find you dribble wee, or are unable to hold your pee? This is because of oestrogen(s) loss that comes with the transition of menopause. You are no longer toned and flexible. Oestrogens also act on the ovaries, vagina, heart, lungs, blood vessels, bone, eyes, breasts and skin, to name but a few.

Oestrogens are the hormones that sing with the woman's body, the hormones that make women women; that make us curvaceous, sexy, shape our breasts, hips, pelvis and even our face. They regulate our menstrual cycle, fertility and, as they plunge drastically, our passage into menopause. Oestrogens prevent migraines related to menstruation. They soften the cervix and produce the vaginal secretion that lubricates during intercourse. They enhance the quality of sexual pleasure. They prevent depression, make us happy, enthusiastic, bouncy and positive. They retard osteoporosis, protect the brain, reduce the risk of heart disease and support the immune system. They increase lean muscle mass and mental and physical vitality, and help maintain a more youthful skin.

Believe it or not, both men and women need oestrogens, but at differing levels. A woman needs higher levels of oestrogens but lower levels of testosterone. A man needs lower levels of oestrogens but higher levels of testosterone.

Contrary to popular belief oestrogens are NOT a single hormone but are made up of a class of many different yet similar oestrogens, the major three being oestrone (E1), oestradiol (E2) and oestriol (E3).

These are primarily secreted by the ovaries, fat cells, muscle cells and skin after menopause. Although the three forms of oestrogens work together, each oestrogen has its own varying activity; this is why they all have different names: (E1) oestrone, (E2) oestradiol and (E3) oestriol.

(E1) Oestrone

Post-menopause, oestrone is the main oestrogen our body produces, and is derived from oestradiol. When levels of E1 are high, we have an increased risk of developing breast and uterine cancer, as it stimulates these tissues.

The only known function of E1 is to act as a reservoir for oestrogens. If our oestrogen(s) levels become too low, our body can steal and use the reserved amount. Pre-menopause, E1 is made in the ovaries, adrenal glands, liver and fat cells, and is converted into E2 in the ovaries. After menopause, or post-menopause, when our ovaries stop working, a very small amount of E1 becomes E2. As time goes on, E1 is made in our fat cells and, to a lesser extent, in our liver and adrenal glands. The more fat accumulation we have, the more E1 we have. This is when it could become risky for overweight women. What happens is, overweight and obese women have an increased oestrone (E1) to oestradiol (E2) ratio, which can lead to an increased risk of breast cancer. Also, we need to avoid frequent alcohol consumption, as this decreases ovarian hormone levels and increases E1. Five nights out a week with the girls, or a drink or two after work to relax you, is not good. I know you like it but think of the consequences before you do it.

(E2) Oestradiol

Oestradiol is the most potent form of oestrogen, being twelve times more potent than E1 (oestrone) and eighty times stronger than E3 (oestriol). This oestrogen in particular 'feminises' the body. It is also responsible for vaginal lubrication, a healthy libido, the female voice and initiating ovulation. E2 helps improve sleep, increases serotonin (a feel-good neurotransmitter), acts as an antioxidant, helps maintain memory, bone and potassium levels, and helps with the absorption of calcium, zinc and magnesium. It increases growth hormone, endorphins (pain-relieving neurotransmitters) and HDL.

E2 (oestradiol) is the main oestrogen our body produces before menopause, the majority of which is produced in the ovaries. High levels of E2 have been associated with an increased risk of developing breast and uterine cancer.

In menopause, E2 is the form of oestrogen we lose due to the slowing down and inactivity of the ovaries as we age, although some postmenopausal women, up to about the age of eighty, do manage to produce a small amount of E2. A hysterectomy, or surgical menopause, affects the levels of E2 to a greater extent than natural menopause, lowering them even further. This is due to the severing and tying off of the uterine artery, which in turn decreases the blood flow to the ovaries.

Some of the symptoms of declining E2 levels in menstruating women include: bladder problems such as infections, more frequent and painful urination and urinary leakage; bone loss resulting in a slumped posture; difficulty achieving orgasm; and decline in collagen levels resulting in the 'haggard look', with more wrinkles and saggy skin; aching joints, muscle soreness and stiffness, increased facial hair, loss of energy, a heavens-the-day-is-long feeling, mood swings, brittle nails, dry eye, fibromyalgia-like pain, food cravings, difficulty in losing weight, anxiety attacks, palpitations (more so prior to menstruation and during) and migraine that is connected to menstruation.

Some of the symptoms I got included restless sleep, especially before a period. That was awful. I suddenly got an allergy and became sensitive to perfumes and chemicals; I had vaginal dryness and pain during intercourse; I became square round my waist and had sudden worsening of PMS. Things I didn't have but many of my friends had and are typical symptoms of declining E2 levels were weight gain, thinning hair and high blood pressure.

(E3) Oestriol

This is the least powerful of the three, although its function is of equal importance. Functions include thickening and humidifying the mucous membranes of the vagina, bladder and eyes, making them resistant to infection. It helps maintain a favourable environment in the gut for the growth of good bacteria. And, here is the big one, it does not promote oestrogen(s)-sensitive cancers such as breast or uterine cancer, but rather protects against them, even when used unopposed, without progesterone (we will talk more about progesterone later).

Oestriol is a by-product of both oestrone and oestradiol metabolism. Oestradiol is converted (made) from testosterone, which can then be converted into oestrone and then back again into oestradiol, like a little storage pot to be used when needed. Oestriol cannot be converted; it is a one-way street.

Oestrogens and the Cancer Influence or Non-Influence Thereof!

Oestrogens have a great influence on the growth or non-growth of breast cell proliferation and possibly cancer. Let me define this for you.

We have two different oestrogen receptors known as ERa (receptor Alpha) and ERb (receptor Beta). Oestrogens that stimulate ERa seem to promote breast cancer proliferation and oestrogens that stimulate ERb inhibit breast cancer proliferation, protecting against breast cancer development. Oestradiol, the stronger one, stimulates ERa and ERb receptors at the same rate or equally, but oestrone is five times more potent in stimulating

ERa vs ERb. This is most likely why high levels of oestrone are seen as being risky in the potential development of breast cancer. Now looking at oestriol is another matter – it stimulates ERb receptors three times more than ERa receptors, which definitely makes breast cancer development less likely. I suppose you could say that oestriol is a type of SERM in its own right (I will tell you more about SERMs in a second), but a good one, a pure one, a safe one, a natural one. One that does not have any nasty side effects, uterine cancer included.

When relatively high doses of oestriol are combined with oestradiol, it inhibits the proliferative effect of these more potent oestrogens (E1 and E2) – basically, it takes up their space by occupying the oestrogen(s) sites in the breast cells. This is far safer than using patentable SERMs and horse hormones.

Patentable SERMs (e.g. tamoxifen and raloxifene) work like this: they compete with oestradiol and oestrone for oestrogen(s) receptor sites, thwarting the actions of these more potent, more carcinogenic oestrogens. But if you remember, they have some bad side effects, such as the worsening of hot flushes and menopausal symptoms, leg cramps, uterine cancer, strokes and blood clots in legs and lungs. Oestriol, on the other hand, has a wide range of oestrogenic effects, such as those mentioned above, along with reducing hot flushes and helping to restore the correct pH of the vagina, which prevents urinary tract infections. E3 does not have the protective qualities E2 has on the brain, bone or heart, although it has been seen to have some positive effects on the heart, helping to lower cholesterol levels.

During pregnancy, oestriol levels rise a thousand fold, safeguarding against maternal breast cancer by counteracting the antagonistic effects of oestradiol. How neat is that? The body really knows what it needs.

Along with the three major oestrogens, there are also about thirty other oestrogens and researchers are continually finding more and different forms.

Something That May Interest You on Synthetic Oestrogens

Synthetic oestrogens, with their many forms of non-human oestrogens, do not fit into the lock-and-key setup in our body. They cannot bind to receptor sites; the key will not open the lock. No one actually knows what happens to the oestrogens that do not fit into our receptor sites. Oestradiol that is produced in our body is easily eliminated through urine within one day, but the synthetic form can take up to thirteen weeks. Our bodies are designed to metabolise our own oestrogens or, in this case, bioidentical hormones that are an exact copy of our own, NOT horse hormones.

Progesterone

Progesterone is a hormone manufactured in the body from the steroid hormone pregnenolone – this is a top-of-the-range hormone synthesised from cholesterol and is a precursor to other sex hormones. Progesterone is primarily produced in the ovaries and adrenal glands, though some is produced in the brain. During pregnancy, it's made in the placenta and becomes dominant, being responsible for the development and survival of the foetus, and for preventing contractions of the uterus and premature birth. Without the correct amounts of progesterone, a pregnancy cannot be successful. Progesterone in women (men have it too) is secreted mostly in the second half of the menstrual cycle, which prevents further ovulation. A thick mucus is produced that is hostile to sperm, preventing passage into the womb. It is responsible for protecting the heart and bones and has an anti-cancer effect, especially against breast cancer and endometrial cancer. It can also help prevent endometriosis.

In 2004, an article in the *International Journal of Cancer* reported that blood levels measured in a group of 5,963 premenopausal women revealed that women with the highest blood levels of progesterone, who had regular menses, experienced an 88% decreased risk of breast cancer. This also confirms another study where 1,083 women who were treated for infertility were then followed for thirty-three years afterwards to determine their subsequent risk of breast cancer. Women deficient in progesterone had a 540% increased risk of premenopausal breast cancer, and were ten times as likely to die from any cancer. For all you ladies out there, the moral of the story is to keep your progesterone levels optimal. Get them checked! It will save your life!

Unlike oestrogens, progesterone is a single molecule. It is both the name and class of this single member, meaning it only has one name, and that would be progesterone not progestin (the latter is a fake, do not get confused). Progesterone has no cousins or relations as oestrogens do. There is not one progesterone that is stronger than the other; there is just one single hormone – pure, natural progesterone. Progesterone receptors are found in an impressive amount of target cells in the body, demonstrating that it has an important effect throughout the body. It is an anabolic steroid, meaning it helps build tissue, creates energy and is essential for growth and repair of body tissue.

Progesterone helps prevent PMS, supports sex drive and is an absolute must for pregnancy and the survival of the foetus. If I had only known that by balancing my progesterone levels with bioidentical progesterone, I could have avoided all those miscarriages. It protects again fibrocystic breasts (fibrocystic breast disease is when a woman has painful and lumpy breasts), restores correct cell oxygen levels, normalises zinc and copper levels, protects again breast and endometrial cancer, facilitates thyroid function, regulates blood sugar levels, stimulates cells for building bone, acts as a natural antidepressant, improves energy, vitality and endurance, and normalises blood clotting. It helps us sleep peacefully, helps our body use and eliminate fats, increases our metabolic rate and promotes a healthy immune system, and our body rids itself of progesterone quickly – unlike progestins. Also, it doesn't cause weight gain as progestins do.

Progesterone does so, so much for us; without it we are lost. Without it we are left with unopposed oestrogen, something which is called 'oestrogen dominance'. This is not a good place to be: it leaves us in a vulnerable situation, defenceless against disease, including cancer. We do not need to get there. We have an option.

Progestins

Progestins, as we already know, are fake progesterone, otherwise called synthetic progesterone, and must never be confused with progesterone or thought of as anything other than a simulation. Progestins are not natural and can cause abnormal menstrual flow or cessation, fluid retention, nausea, insomnia, jaundice, depression, fever, weight fluctuation, allergic reactions and development of male characteristics. As synthetic progesterone is foreign to the body and does not have the full range of biological activity compared with natural progesterone, it causes problems and has actually been shown to inhibit biosynthesis (production) of progesterone. Our body really has a big problem with metabolising alien hormones. Metabolise means to chemically change, neutralise and/or dispose of the hormone. When an alien hormone is introduced, the body metabolises it differently, finding it confusing and creating toxic by-products. Endogenous or bioidentical hormones are, on the other hand, read perfectly.

Example:
Taking the pill or oral contraceptive at an early age (teens) is a known risk factor for breast cancer. The sooner a girl begins the higher her risk is. In fact, girls that take the pill between the ages of thirteen to eighteen have a 600% increased chance of getting breast cancer. This would be due to the progestins (fake progesterone) in the birth control pill that interfere with the beneficial actions of natural progesterone, and also because ovulation is blocked (anovulation), therefore stopping the production of the ovaries' natural hormones, including oestrogens.

Apart from interfering with the body's own production of progesterone, once progestins are in the body they can attach to many of the body's receptor sites, and not only progesterone receptors. In other words, everything just goes haywire, putting us at risk. Tell your daughter, granddaughter, the neighbour's daughter too – everyone.

Oestrogens and Progesterone

We already know that hormones work together in symphony, each being part of a large, intricate network of various systems, hormones and metabolic mediators. This is particularly true of oestrogens and progesterone – it is important that these two groups of hormones remain at a specific ratio within our body. It's like teamwork, despite the fact that their roles appear to be on opposite sides of the net: if one moves without the other then problems may arise and certainly an imbalance will occur. The fact is that it is the resulting effect of these two groups of hormones that help balance each other out and keeps them functioning correctly. We should never be encouraged to take oestrogens exclusively as it is the balancing effect of progesterone that protects us from such things as heart disease and oestrogen(s)-sensitive cancers, among other things.

Here's something else that may interest you. E2 increases insulin sensitivity and improves glucose tolerance, while progesterone decreases insulin sensitivity and can cause insulin resistance. So, all you women out there who have diabetes, it is *even more important* for you to ensure that your oestrogens/progesterone ratio is within these norms. Other side effects of high progesterone to low oestrogens are decreased sexual interest, fatigue, and with it along comes depression.

A ratio with too much progesterone will create a breakdown of protein and muscle, which in turn will make diseases like fibromyalgia (which is classed as an autoimmune disease and makes our muscles hurt like hell) worse.

Oestrogen Dominance

In perimenopause both oestrogens and progesterone levels drop; oestrogens by 40% to 60%, and progesterone levels can drop to nearly zero. Usually, progesterone declines first. What this means is that a woman may have excessive, normal or deficient oestrogen(s) levels only because progesterone levels drop so drastically, which creates an imbalance or the so-called 'oestrogen dominance effect', even though oestrogen(s) levels are not excessively high. In other words, the term 'oestrogen dominance' doesn't necessarily mean we have too many oestrogens; it means we don't have enough progesterone. We have an imbalance.

Oestrogens such as E2 (oestradiol) and E1 (oestrone) are promoters of cell growth, being firstly responsible for the message that encourages the growth of the blood-rich tissue in the uterus in the first half of the menstrual cycle in preparation for implantation of the fertilised egg. It is this function (cell growth) that potentially makes oestrogen dominance (or lack of progesterone) a dangerous promoter of cancer. One of progesterone's jobs is to keep oestrogens' growth-promoting status in check, keeping cell growth in balance and protecting against oestrogen(s)-sensitive cancers such as uterine and breast cancer. If this does not occur we are in trouble: we get oestrogen dominance. We need progesterone to counteract the antagonistic effects of oestrogens.

Progesterone helps prevent oestrogen(s)-sensitive cancers in two ways. Firstly, by reducing the number of oestrogen(s) receptors in such places as the uterine lining or breast. When oestrogen(s) receptors are prevented from binding or attaching themselves to a site (e.g. uterus or breast) because of progesterone, they cannot then stimulate cell growth. The second reason is that progesterone directly regulates cell division or replication of mature oestrogen(s)-sensitive cells, blocking oestrogen(s)-stimulated cellular overgrowth, and therefore cancer.

Oestrogen dominance may lead to a hysterectomy, which should not happen and need not happen. The only circumstances under which it should happen is if there is cancer. No other single reason should be given, especially in this day and age. When we are oestrogen dominant we get a continual build-up of the uterus lining (endometrium) which becomes so thick it will eventually cause breakthrough bleeding, or even haemorrhaging. This is what happened to my mother. Of course, doctors didn't know any better in those days, so we can forgive them. But the doctors of today that continue to offer this way out cannot be forgiven. There is no need! It really makes me angry, I mean, come on, let's be a bit more imaginative about this. Why take out a body part that we need, why not correct the symptom, a symptom that is screaming at us? It can be done. Why not cycle the correct ratios of oestrogens and progesterone into the woman's body and correct this symptom? Our body is telling us we have an imbalance that needs to be corrected. By doing a hysterectomy, these doctors are only covering up the symptom that is waiting to be heard to an even louder degree. By covering up, the worst is yet to come. This is when cancer cells have the opportunity to grow and proliferate. Our body is talking to us. We should listen to what it is saying.

Oestrogen dominance may also occur in younger women when there is lack of ovulation (anovulation). In a young woman's cycle an egg is released usually from days twelve to fourteen when oestrogens are at their peak. Once the egg is released it travels from the ovaries through the fallopian tube to the uterus in preparation for fertilisation. When ovulation does not occur, progesterone is not produced in any significant amounts, giving way to oestrogen dominance. A premenopausal woman may still have a normal menstrual cycle even if she has not ovulated. She could then experience PMS symptoms such as swollen and tender breasts, weight gain, mood swings and cramps. When oestrogen dominance does occur in younger women and they start feeling an imbalance, sometimes they can be given progesterone exclusively, as they already have enough oestrogens. This will help to put things back into balance.

While we are on the subject, you may be interested to know that low progesterone levels have been implicated in postpartum depression. Luckily, and once again, this can be rectified by restoring and balancing the body with bioidentical hormones until Mummy starts feeling like herself again. Once the baby is born (naturally or by C-section) and the umbilical cord is cut, our oestrogen(s) levels drop two thousand times more than the drop we experience before our menstrual cycle begins. At the same time our progesterone levels also fall abruptly.

After a pregnancy our body resets its hormone levels. If the mother is unable to immediately rev up production of progesterone, she will then be left in a total state of hormonal imbalance, which may bring about postpartum depression, and she certainly will not be feeling good in herself. It happened to me. I didn't want to see my first boy, Jonathan, immediately after the birth although, at the same time, I felt terribly guilty – and yet, didn't want to see him. I did not understand. I do now. My hormones were askew. It was not my fault. Although mine was the 'baby blues', rather than the more severe symptoms of postpartum depression, which last longer.

Unfortunately, so many of these poor mums are just handed antidepressants and sent off with a pat on their back to get on with it. Antidepressants are drugs and can create a false sense of security, and certainly do not put back what is missing, or resolve the problem. Just balancing hormones can do that. Really, is it that difficult? Our body does not produce antidepressants, so does not have and will never have a deficiency of this chemical drug. Our body is telling us that we need to restore the hormones that, in some cases, cannot be sufficiently produced after pregnancy.

Thyroid hormone levels can also be dysfunctional directly after delivery, which may cause postpartum thyroid disorders. Postpartum thyroid disorders can also occur up to three years after delivery. 5–10% of women may suffer from postpartum thyroid disorders. Since symptoms of oestrogens and/or progesterone loss are similar to those of an underactive thyroid (hypothyroidism), we definitely need an expert in restorative medicine to check in with.

As you will have understood, progesterone has a balancing effect on oestrogens but the ratio between oestrogens and progesterone has to be correct. Only an experienced doctor practising restorative medicine can help you find this ratio, but you need to be patient as the perfecting of ratios can take time. Careful dosing and hormone level monitoring are an essential factor in the correct practice of restorative medicine. More often than not (I would say always), this is ignored or not even considered in HRT regimes. The way HRT has been handed out to women is mind-boggling. It does not resemble nature in any way. Firstly, progesterone in nature does not flow every day as it does in the form of a drug conjugated from horse oestrogens and progestin. Nor is it compatible with what we make in our own body. They are alien hormones that have no right to be there. They confuse our brain and because of this, as we already know, have terrible side effects, one of which is cancer. The rule of the day is play safe. Go and restore your body with bioidentical hormones!

Excess oestrogens are the culprit for PMS, night sweats and depression. They also seem to create a deficiency in zinc, magnesium and vitamins B6, C and A. These are all important to the maintenance of a healthy hormonal balance. Magnesium is extremely important in warding off heart attacks.

Oestrogen dominance (or progesterone deficiency) causes a long list of symptoms, some of which are: anxiety, decreased sex drive, depression, decreased HDL levels, weight gain, pain and inflammation, nervousness, osteoporosis, hypersensitivity, insomnia, excessive menstruation (heavy bleeding that lasts more than seven days), mood swings, irritability and migraines prior to menstruation – I now understand why so many of my friends suffered from migraines and developed breast cancer.

Some of the causes of oestrogen dominance or low progesterone can be due to antidepressant drugs, high sugar intake, stress, decreased thyroid hormone, low luteinising hormone (LH) and an increase in prolactin production. Prolactin is the hormone of nursing mothers; it decreases ovarian hormone production after delivery, which helps protect against a new pregnancy while still nursing. There is also an excess or increased production of prolactin in menopause.

Other Causes of Oestrogen Dominance

As there are so many oestrogens in our everyday lives due to pesticides, plastics, industrial waste products, car exhaust, meat, soaps, furniture, carpets, panelling and insulation in offices and houses, it tends to cause oestrogen dominance. These oestrogens are called xenoestrogens and are capable of mimicking oestrogens in our body as they all have some form of oestrogenic activity. The most notable sources of chemical oestrogens are petroleum-based products, pollutants, pesticides, herbicides, fungicides and plastics. Definitely don't drink out of plastic bottles.

Testosterone

'The male hormone' – here we go again. But we know better, don't we? We know what balanced levels of testosterone can do for our bodies as well. Testosterone falls into a class of hormones called androgens, all known as 'male hormones'. Androgens include testosterone, DHEA, DHEA-S, androstenediol and androstenedione. Testosterone and androstenedione can act as precursors for the manufacture of oestradiol and oestrone, which is very important for postmenopausal women because, by this time, their ovaries have stopped producing oestradiol.

As hormones decline with age, sexuality also declines. Oestrogens and progesterone are significant in maintaining women's organs, keeping them healthy and in good working order, keeping vaginal tissue thick, lubricated and free from infections, and helping us to enjoy pain-free intercourse. However, oestrogens do not have any direct effect on libido, whereas testosterone and the other androgens (androstenedione, androstenediol, DHEA and DHEA-S) do, being mainly responsible for charging the batteries of sexual desire, encouraging enjoyment, fantasy and orgasm. With low testosterone levels, sex becomes a chore. "Does he really want it again?!" Add 'a touch of love' by adding bioidentical testosterone to improve quality of sex and orgasm. Testosterone stimulates love and affection, as well as sexual emotions.

Women have testosterone levels one-tenth to one-twelfth of those of men. Levels start declining as far back as a woman's late twenties and thirties, mainly due to the age-related drop in the testosterone precursor DHEA. The decline not only starts earlier for us than men but, initially, at a greater rate. A twenty-year-old woman has approximately double the amount of testosterone that a forty-year-old one has. We naturally have a high oestrogens to low testosterone ratio. Men, on the other hand, have a high testosterone to low oestrogens ratio. Nature has decided that for us. It's the ratio that differentiates men from women, it's part of life, nature; *Songs in the Key of Life.* When that ratio is out, in either men or women, we spiral into a decline. It is the ratio between the two that keeps us looking and feeling good.

Testosterone is produced in the adrenal glands and ovaries. A woman's body metabolises testosterone into oestrogens. During and after menopause when oestrogens and progesterone suddenly nosedive and the ovaries start to shrivel up and eventually cease the secretion of oestradiol (and progesterone), testosterone secretion is independent of this and continues its steady decline that began twenty to thirty years earlier, following through with age.

Testosterone is an important factor in our behaviour and our look. Women with low testosterone levels will be less inclined to go to the gym, will be less motivated do any physical movement and certainly will be more passive. Be warned, women taking the birth control pill will have lower levels of testosterone: what happens is that the ovaries take time off and then the woman becomes more dependent on the adrenals and the production of DHEA for her testosterone. Remember DHEA is also made in the adrenals and is the precursor to oestrogens and testosterone.

Just let me sidetrack for a second and talk a little about men. It is, of course, important for them to have balanced levels of testosterone too. Testosterone is needed for erection, ejaculation and fertility. A man is incapable of erection when oestrogens outweigh testosterone; the ratio then becomes high oestrogens to low testosterone. This is the time when the diseases of ageing start to become apparent: almost every disease starts with a hormonal decline in both men and women. Interestingly, over the last twenty years, men's average testosterone levels have dropped by 16%. Frightening – I really think we should reconsider the way we live our lives.

I would be discrediting testosterone if I were only to mention its sexual power. Testosterone is an anabolic steroid, and a plus-plus hormone. It helps build muscle mass and strength, reduces body fat and helps increase muscle tone. Testosterone relieves fatigue and ups our flagging energy levels. Many of my friends complain about lack of stamina and get-up-and-go. Testosterone lessens depression and the risk of osteoporosis, and improves symptoms of diabetes and high cholesterol.

Low levels of testosterone may result in low self-esteem and lack of confidence, saggy cheeks, varicose veins, cellulite, fat accumulation in the breast and abdomen (weight gain), dry, thin skin with poor elasticity, muscle wasting, hypersensitive and hyperemotional states, thin lips and loss of pubic hair. They may also dream less.

Low testosterone has also been associated with Alzheimer's disease. Testosterone acts directly on neurons (nerve cells) in the brain, as do progesterone and oestrogens, helping to increase connections between neurons. It also protects neurons from being attacked by neurotoxins and free radicals, and enhances vasodilation and blood flow in the brain. In other words testosterone, progesterone and oestrogens protect the brain and may protect against the loss of memory and cognition we see in perimenopause and menopause, as well as the progression of Alzheimer's and dementia. To have a youthful, muscular body we need optimal amounts of testosterone. No point going to the gym every day, slogging your heart out trying to achieve the body you've always dreamed of, when you ain't got enough testosterone – it just won't happen. The ratio and balance is important. Testosterone rebuilds bone by stimulating the formation of new bone; it improves tissue oxygenation, and strengthens and protects the heart by nurturing the cardiac muscle – which, by the way, has more testosterone receptor sites than any other muscle in the body, so testosterone keeps our heart strong and pumping efficiently.

As with other hormones, we can have too much testosterone in the body, which may be due to overconsumption of sugar and carbohydrates. When we hit menopause and our passage into it, about 20% of us will have high testosterone levels that will not decline with age. Unless, of course, we restore our body. To acquire optimal health, the replacement and regulation of the amount of testosterone we need throughout our life is key. For testosterone to work at its best, oestradiol (E2) also needs to be optimised. When there are not enough oestrogens present, testosterone cannot attach to our brain receptors, which in turn dictates how well testosterone works in our body.

Some symptoms of excess testosterone may include facial hair. You know those older women you see walking around with moustaches? They have a hormonal imbalance. I remember my gran used to shave hers. I walked in on her one day when she was shaving; she was so embarrassed, poor thing. I will never forget her face; my heart sank for her. Other symptoms include fatigue, fluid retention, hair loss, anger, agitation, acne or oily skin, depression, changes in memory, increased risk of developing breast cancer, poor prognosis if we have breast cancer, weight gain, infertility, mood swings, irregular periods and increased insulin resistance. Polycystic ovary syndrome

(PCOS) is also another symptom of high testosterone. This is mainly due to an adrenal imbalance which occurs in younger women.

Going back to men again, grumpy men, with well-rounded bellies, shrinking muscles and downturned mouths are also displaying signs of a decline in testosterone levels. Men who hide themselves away, don't like going out and have lost their vitality and verve are on the rocky road to disease. This theory/story that testosterone replacement causes cancer is a myth. In fact, it is the exact opposite: restoring what has been lost will give them back their life. There is no clinical evidence that the risk of either prostate cancer or BPH (benign prostatic hyperplasia) increases with testosterone replacement therapy. When men's hormone levels decline they see a rise in prostate specific antigen (PSA), and along comes the risk of prostate cancer. When men restore their hormone levels to optimal, they will notice that their energy levels return and their verve for life reignites. They will look better, feel better, they will build muscle and that 'grumpy-old-man syndrome' will be gone. The drug Lupron, which is the equivalent of tamoxifen for women, has terrible debilitating effects. Lupron messes with hormones. It works by shutting off hormones in the brain and deactivating the signal needed to make hormones. It is chemical castration! Quality of life is zero and there is an increased risk of diabetes and heart disease. Who wants to get there? Restoring missing testosterone to youthful levels does not stimulate cancer. The benefits of fully restoring the body will protect their hearts and brains, and has an astounding ability to prevent cancer.

DHEA: Dehydroepiandrosterone

DHEA is the most prevalent steroid hormone in the human body and one of the most essential hormones in human health. In fact, with few exceptions, low or deficient DHEA is found in every illness. It is considered an important restorative hormone

Women produce approximately 30% less than men, which may be why women seem to be more affected by adrenal stress than men. Women's ovaries contribute a small amount to DHEA production, along with the brain and skin, but mostly the adrenal gland is responsible for production. DHEA is at its highest level, optimal, at about age twenty-five, and its levels are more than ten times higher than those of any other hormone in the body. This fact shows that it must be there for a good reason. Thereafter, it declines steadily, as a function of age, and by the time we hit fifty there is a minimal amount compared to the amount we had in the heydays of our twenties. Post-menopause, nearly all oestrogens created in a woman's body are produced from the conversion via DHEA.

Although men produce higher levels of DHEA than women, because a significant amount is produced in the testes as well as the adrenal, their age-related decline of DHEA is more drastic than ours and, by the age of seventy, they have roughly equal amounts to women. Optimal levels of DHEA protect both male and female from cardiovascular disease, although it doesn't have such a dramatic effect as testosterone.

DHEA is a major marker for age and health. It can be converted into various hormones (derivatives), including testosterone and oestradiol. It is because of these derivatives that DHEA is such a powerful and important restorative hormone. One important benefit, among many, is that it stabilises the negative effects of excess cortisol (I discuss this further in the Adrenal Fatigue section).

DHEA has positive effects on the immune system, brain, muscle and reproductive organs, keeps mucous membranes moist and soft, boosts energy, promotes hair growth and fights anxiety, depression, diabetes, liver disease and cancer. It slows osteoporosis and increases bone mass, improves insulin resistance and helps wounds to heal at a greater speed. It also aids older women in getting pregnant. DHEA is used as an additional therapy for treating female infertility, along with natural progesterone. It has also been shown to reduce the symptoms of systemic lupus erythematosus, and even helps maintain collagen levels in the skin. A French study known as the DHEAge Study noted that DHEA supplementation greatly improved skin tone, colour, thickness and hydration.

Women with hormone-receptive breast cancer should always get advice from a doctor qualified in restorative medicine before supplementing with DHEA. DHEA-derived oestrogens may have the same risk-increasing effects as any other oestrogens on the breast, if not monitored correctly. Always, always get advice and blood tests done – supplementing with any hormones requires monitoring by a qualified restorative doctor. The balance and ratios have to be correct.

Let me explain the difference between DHEA and DHEA-S (DHEA-sulphate), just to save confusion. These two values are used to measure DHEA levels. DHEA-S is a metabolite of DHEA and can be converted back to DHEA, its precursor. There is much more DHEA-S found in the blood, so it provides a much better gauge of how much DHEA we have in the body.

Pregnenolone: the First Port of Call

I take all the above mentioned hormones, and others, including pregnenolone. My concentration, thinking power, memory and quality of life have improved greatly since reinstating my life, as yours will too. I intend to stay internally young and keep disease out of my life by continuing this regime.

Pregnenolone decreases with age, as with all hormones. At age seventy-five we have approximately 65% less than we had when we were thirty-five.

Pregnenolone is manufactured in the adrenal glands. The adrenal glands produce a cascade of hormones which include progesterone, DHEA, testosterone, oestrogens, aldosterone and cortisol. All these hormones are derived from a substance called cholesterol, which is made up of its own specific building blocks; a complex procedure that I will explain later. Cholesterol then converts into pregnenolone, which is known as the 'grandmother hormone' because the body converts it into all of the other adrenal hormones (except adrenaline and noradrenaline). Progesterone and DHEA are next to be produced.

As pregnenolone, DHEA and progesterone occur at the beginning of the adrenal cascade, it allows our body to decide which other hormones the body needs at a specific time. The body is very intelligent. When pregnenolone is used together with other sex hormones such as oestrogens, progesterone, testosterone and DHEA, an inferior dose of these hormones can be used and it is found to be less physiologically disturbing. Everything has to be in balance for the song of life to play well.

Pregnenolone taken in the morning promotes good sleep and improves the deep, dreamless stage of sleep called delta-wave sleep. If pregnenolone is taken in the evening, it can have the opposite effect and cause insomnia, as the brain continues to work. As we age, the amount of deep sleep we get declines and, as we know, nothing happens in the body without consequence. Diminished delta-wave sleep lowers melatonin levels and growth hormone production, which brings about premature ageing.

Pregnenolone is found in the brain in high concentrations and it not only helps us cope with stress, it enhances concentration, improves memory and is a key player in mood control. If we are under persistent or long-term stress, our levels of pregnenolone drop and so, subsequently, do all the other adrenal hormones (we will talk more about this later), including the sex hormones, which act as a natural antioxidant that helps prevent oxidative damage caused by cortisol. Oxidative damage is one of the major reasons for accelerated ageing. We need to keep our sex hormone levels optimal because the lower they are, the more damage they cause to tissue, and more so when we are under stress.

Pregnenolone is not only a precursor to other steroid hormones, it also belongs to a group called neurosteroids, as do DHEA and progesterone. Neurosteroids are important for regulating the balance between excitation and inhibition of neurons in the nervous system. OK, so you are not sure what that means. Neurons communicate, they shoot out messages via both chemicals and electricity. These messages and impulses travel along the nervous system at breakneck speed. Neurons are responsible for our daily functions that enable us to live. Movement: lifting our arm up and down, walking in the park, closing the fridge door. Being able to respond to a stimulus on time and react to impulses promptly is pretty important in life, but being able to control this excitability is just as important. Low levels of pregnenolone have been associated with dementia in elderly patients. Alzheimer's disease is the most common form of dementia.

A decrease in pregnenolone causes symptoms such as feeling tired, being unable to cope with stress and having a lack of the energy and enthusiasm we once had. Other signs of below-optimal levels include low blood pressure, joint pains, frequent urination, cravings for salty foods, a loss of underarm and pubic hair and increased risk of infections.

Supplementing with bioidentical pregnenolone, when there is a deficiency, helps stimulate concentration and clarify thinking, prevents memory loss, fights depression, relieves arthritis and speeds healing.

Melatonin

With melatonin the decline starts just after the age of fifteen. By the time we double on that and reach thirty, we produce less than half of our youthful levels and, by the time we double up again and reach sixty, we are producing less than one tenth of what we had in our youth. It is secreted by the pineal gland and very small amounts are produced in the retina and GI tract. Its secretion is increased by the darkness but inhibited by light, natural or artificial. That is why we begin to feel tired as night falls and we wake up when dawn approaches. Even the smallest pinpoint of light during the night can lower levels of melatonin production.

When we are asleep, the electrical activity of our brain is slow and interspersed with moments associated with dreaming. Without sufficient melatonin we will get a poor quality of sleep that is deprived of dreams and full of agitation. When we are awake, the electrical activity of our brain is highly active. In sleep, our blood pressure drops, our breathing becomes slower and the body's metabolism also slows. For a healthy brain and body, all of these changes are essential. Without sleep, we cannot be healthy.

Sweet dreams are what we need for our brain and our body, and this is where melatonin steps in. Melatonin is a potent sleep hormone. Remember, sleep is one of our greatest healers. It regenerates the brain and every other part of the body. Melatonin regulates our sleep-wake cycle, the circadian rhythm that is so important to our body's equilibrium. It talks to other hormones that rise and fall within this twenty-four hour cycle and sets our internal biological clock. Stress, ageing and travel affect sleep patterns and in turn will affect melatonin levels.

As melatonin declines, our immune system also declines, and things start going wrong as the immune system begins to malfunction. We're in trouble. We need to protect against age-related diseases. Melatonin is a potent antioxidant and is a key player in the modulation of the immune system. Melatonin has an incredible revitalising effect on the immune system, kind of waking it up, helping to protect against breast cancer and all cancers generally. A woman's lifetime risk of developing any form of cancer is one to three, and one to eight for breast cancer. Melatonin directly blocks cancer cell proliferation (multiplication and growth) and at the same time, increases the tumour-suppressor genes (p53 and p21); it reduces the concentration of oestrogen(s) receptor alpha (ER alpha), therefore reducing the stimulating effects of oestradiol on cancer cells in the breast.

Melatonin affects the hypothalamus and the pituitary glands, and influences nearly all the other hormones in the body, along with the thymus gland, which is central to the development and correct functioning of our immune system. As melatonin declines, the thymus shrinks and, by the time we are sixty, it has almost disappeared. Anything that upholds the integrity of the immune system should uphold us. Apart from supporting the immune system, melatonin plays other important roles including neuroprotection and anti-inflammatory defence – inflammation promotes cancer, among other things.

Melatonin has so many beneficial effects on our body, from bone health and obesity to heart disease and diabetes, and may also protect our genetic material.

Halting free radical damage with the use of antioxidants is part of restorative medicine's regime. Melatonin is, as mentioned earlier, a powerful antioxidant and defends the body against free radical cell damage, which protects against free radical-related diseases such as cardiovascular disease, cancer and so many other age-related diseases in between. Melatonin possesses 200% more antioxidant power than vitamin E and is superior to glutathione as well as vitamins C and E in reducing oxidative damage. And it doesn't stop there: there is an increased production of the naturally occurring antioxidants inside our cells, such as glutathione. Melatonin is one of the few antioxidants that enter into the nucleus of all the cells and protect the DNA. By doing this, it not only prevents cancer but also helps delay the onset of many neurodegenerative diseases such as Alzheimer's disease, Parkinson's disease and Huntington's disease.

Melatonin improves the function of mitochondria and helps to protect them from oxidative damage and decay. The decline in mitochondria is a major player of many neurodegenerative diseases including the above mentioned. Mitochondria are the centre of our cells and are energy-generating motors; all life functions are dependent on the energetic fuel produced in the mitochondria, which is called ATP (adenosine triphosphate). Unfortunately, as with everything in life, this incredible power-generating system deteriorates with age, producing less energy and allowing more free radicals to escape – another reason why optimal levels of melatonin are so important. And, ladies, melatonin affects the release of sex hormones. Everything in the body is interrelated.

Supplementing with melatonin is not only important, it is a must. It is an anti-cancer hormone, a natural anti-ageing molecule, a major free-radical scavenger – an overall star. Many other free radical and age-related diseases such as macular degeneration, acute respiratory distress syndrome (ARDS), glaucoma and sepsis have all been responsive to increased levels of melatonin.

My grandmother had age-related macular degeneration, as did my mother. I am not looking forward to going blind! I take melatonin every single night, along with my other hormones, and while I sleep peacefully, I let the antioxidant effect fight the battle for life and sight.

Melatonin is an aromatase inhibitor that blocks the production of oestradiol from testosterone, which is particularly good for men. You already know about the dangers of an imbalance of oestrogens to testosterone in men – they don't want too many oestrogens. As men get older, they convert more testosterone into oestradiol, more so if they are fatter as conversion takes place in fat. Let's keep the muscle strong, the fat off and disease out.

Melatonin is made from the amino acid tryptophan, which is used to make the brain chemical serotonin. When melatonin levels go up, serotonin levels fall. If we eat too many sugary carbohydrates, we make less melatonin mainly because carbohydrates cause a shift in amino acid balance to make more serotonin.

Melatonin, serotonin and dopamine are all potent brain chemicals. Both serotonin and dopamine are neurotransmitters. Melatonin is a hormone, a neurotransmitter, but not a steroid hormone. A neurotransmitter is a chemical messenger that carries and modulates (regulates) signals between nerve cells (neurons) and other cells in the body.

Serotonin is the brain's feel-good neurotransmitter. This is the chemical that keeps us happy and the brain jumping with joy. Serotonin activity is essential for keeping us dancing in kitchen while preparing dinner. It is a neurotransmitter that talks directly to the enjoyment centre of our brain.

Although serotonin is produced in the brain, where it performs profound functions, some 95% is found in our intestines, where it plays a major role in modulating the perception of pain and regulating secretions and movement in the intestines, helping the normal function of the digestive system. As with all good things in life, serotonin declines with age. Abnormal serotonin metabolism has been associated with many health problems such as migraine, cluster headaches, anorexia, bulimia, anxiety, bodily aches, yeast infections, foggy thinking, insomnia, depression and gut disturbances, due to faulty communication between serotonin in the gut, and the brain and spinal cord. This is your gut feeling coming out.

Dopamine is responsible for many things, but I like to call it the 'reward hormone'. Dopamine levels decrease significantly with age; that is why we cannot enjoy music to the extent we once did. Sad life. Do you remember when we used to listen to a favourite song, blasting it out so everyone could hear? The sheer enjoyment of it all? What happens is that when we hear this wonderful music, the brain releases larger amounts of dopamine than normal and our levels rise, giving us a sense of peaceful satisfaction and reward! Age takes this away from us; life just isn't like it once was. So unfair. That is what I had lost: my love of life, my dopamine and serotonin input, and my hormones.

Female hormones are powerful modulators and greatly affect the brain chemicals, serotonin, dopamine and GABA. When there is an imbalance of female hormones there will also be an imbalance of the electrical activity of our brain. To give you an example, when we have low E2, we will have low serotonin. You see, it is all interrelated; the body is just one big network that keeps talking to itself. We need to restore our body. We need balance.

GABA (gamma-aminobutyric acid) is a part of the brain system that allows us to manage our moods, thoughts and actions, so is critical to how we think and act. GABA is our braking system. Other neurotransmitters provide the sparks and petrol, exciting the brain; GABA on the other hand is a neurotransmitter that relaxes and calms our brain and inhibits excessive activity, which, for example, in depression can result in excessive negative thinking.

Note: Serotonin taken orally is unable to cross the blood-brain barrier. What is the blood-brain barrier, you may ask? Simply put, it is the division between the blood circulating in our bodies from the fluid surrounding our brain. This is the brain's safeguard. It keeps the invaders out, such as bacteria and large molecules, but at the same time, allows in such things as oxygen and hormones that are required by the brain. As orally-taken serotonin does not cross the blood-brain barrier, 5-HTP (5-Hydroxytryptophan) would be prescribed, which is a precursor of serotonin (and melatonin) that can cross the blood-brain barrier.

Thyroid

The thyroid is a very significant gland and found in the lower part of the neck, just below the Adam's apple. It releases the iodine-containing hormones (thyroid hormones), thyroxine (T4) and triiodothyronine (T3), and regulates the body's metabolism, temperature and heart rate. Functions of the thyroid gland include tissue repair and development, aiding the function of mitochondria, controlling hormone excretion and oxygen utilisation, regulating vitamin usage, assisting in the digestion process, regulating growth and stimulating protein synthesis.

Thyroid function is very complex and profoundly affects nearly every other organ in the body. Therefore, the body and its systems are dependent on the correct functioning of the thyroid gland. When thyroid function declines, so does the immune system. When the immune system's reaction is slow, microbes have time to multiply and proliferate – we want to get these microbes out of our system as soon as possible. All cells in the body communicate with each other and every cell in the body is affected by the thyroid as it controls the speed at which energy is used by the cells.

To understand thyroid function is to understand yourself. To understand that joint pain, allergies, carpal tunnel syndrome, high insulin, high cholesterol, fibrocystic breast disease (noncancerous changes in the breast tissue), unexplained weight gain, hair loss, decreased sex drive and many more complaints are correlated to low thyroid. When there is a thyroid dysfunction you just won't feel good. That is how I felt. At the time I just could not put my finger on it, but I know now. Like I said, mornings were slow and nights deprived of sleep made me feel even worse. Mornings at the gym were hard to bear. I could not manage to do the workouts I had once done. I knew it was more than just my age, that there was something more behind it. Those doctors; they were so wrong. To feel good, the thyroid must function at optimum. That's just the way it is. We do not want too much thyroid nor too little, as with all hormones. When the thyroid gland dysfunctions, it can either produce too much thyroid, which is known as hyperthyroidism, or too little thyroid, known as hypothyroidism.

In menopause it is common for thyroid problems to appear – that's where my problems came from. With the decline of oestradiol and progesterone, along with testosterone from our ovaries, it effects the thyroid and may leave us with a 'go-slow' thyroid. Our ovaries have thyroid receptors and our thyroid gland has receptors for oestrogens and progesterone. It makes sense that something is going to 'hit the fan'.

There are a few types of thyroid hormones that are produced in the body. Let's take a brief look at how the thyroid works. Thyroid-stimulating hormone (TSH) is made in the pituitary gland. Thyroxine (T4) and Triiodothyronine (T3) are made in the thyroid gland. T3 is the active hormone and T4 is the inactive hormone, being 80% of the thyroid gland's production. Our body has to change or convert T4 into T3. We have no T4 receptors in our body, only T3 receptors.

The thyroid functions through the pituitary gland and the hypothalamus. These highly functioning organs stay tuned to how much T4 is circulating in the blood. When there is a decrease of T4 levels the pituitary gland then secretes thyroid-stimulating hormone (TSH), which stimulates the thyroid to produce more T4. Because of this relayed message, thyroxine in the blood increases and, naturally, the production of TSH is then quelled, as TSH no longer needs to stimulate. This is what is called a feedback loop, and functions to maintain a constant level of thyroid hormone in the body.

Once T4 is circulating in the blood the conversion into the active form T3 takes place. In times of long-term mental and physical stress, or when dieting and trying to lose weight, the conversion of T4 into T3 is affected. And, of course, we had to get to this point – age! With age the production of T4 decreases and, of course, without doubt, the conversion of T4 to T3 also declines. What happens? Cell-to-cell information is not fully received. The transfer message is interrupted, resulting in the body not working at optimum. This is when the symptoms of hypothyroid become apparent.

The thing is, most doctors don't get this; they do not know how to test for hypothyroidism. I expect – well, I know, really – that this is what happened to me. When we go for thyroid tests, the entire thyroid panel should be measured. This includes total T4, total T3, free T3, reverse T3, free T4, TSH and thyroid antibodies (if our antibodies are too high, they can stop the thyroid hormone binding to the thyroid receptors, then obviously we get symptoms of low thyroid function). Conventional doctors only test T4. Now how on earth can we expect to get the correct results if they are doing less than half the job? Without a full panel (full blood tests) we will not get a precise reading and we will, like me, be left with symptoms that totally disrupt our life. So unfair, and it's so easy to correct in the end.

Reverse T3 is the opposite of T3; it only has 1% of the activity that T3 does. The higher the levels of reverse T3 are, the lower the levels of T3 will be, mainly because both these T3s bind to the same receptor sites, meaning that they cannot both occupy the same sites simultaneously. If there is a high reverse T3, T3 will not be able to do its job correctly. The name given to high reverse T3 levels is 'reverse T3 dominance'. When this happens, we can get all the symptoms of 'go-slow' thyroid (hypothyroidism), including weight gain. When reverse T3 levels remain elevated, it is very difficult to lose weight and keep it off, which can be very discouraging and depressing. Make sure you get a full panel done or you will be a very, very unhappy person, with weight gain to go with it.

Stress is the most common reason reverse T3 becomes high. We will talk a lot about stress in the following pages but, for now, I will just tell you that stress causes cortisol to rise. Cortisol is a hormone. Long-term stress causes cortisol to stay high, which may cause your body to secrete more reverse T3. Other causes of reverse T3 include autoimmune disease, hormonal imbalances, infections, exposure to environmental toxins (chemical pollutants, pesticides, mercury, fluoride – fluoride blocks iodine binding), food deprivation, poor liver function and nutritional deficiencies.

When there is a decreased production of T3 (and higher levels of reverse T3), it can cause cholesterol levels to increase; this is because when there are low levels of T3, less cholesterol will be transported out of the blood, which causes an increase in the so-called 'bad' cholesterol (we will talk more about cholesterol later on).

As I stated previously, hypothyroidism is when too little thyroid is being produced. Something to think about is that 25% of perimenopausal women have some kind of thyroid problem (that is because something hit the fan). In most cases this is due to subclinical hypothyroidism which may progress into overt hypothyroidism. Both subclinical and overt hypothyroidism should be treated. Subclinical hypothyroidism is most commonly an early stage of hypothyroidism. Overt hypothyroidism is usually diagnosed round about age sixty, post-menopause, and its prevalence is increased with age. It is estimated that one in five women and one in ten men over sixty suffer from underactive thyroids.

Subclinical hypothyroidism was what I was finally diagnosed with. I could have gone to my GP or gynaecologist forever and it would never have been discovered. God knows what state I would have been in by now. Fat, tired, very slow-moving, very unhappy and definitely not so healthy. This is when it is important that you go to an expert in restorative medicine. Many cases of midlife hypothyroidism are caused by oestrogen dominance. When the oestrogens-to-progesterone ratio is high, it can block the action of thyroid hormone so, even when the thyroid gland is producing normal levels of the hormone, it becomes ineffective and we get symptoms of hypothyroidism. As the thyroid gland itself is functioning correctly, when a thyroid test is done, it may show normal thyroid levels in our system, although we have the classic symptoms. What I am saying is that thyroid function is so complex and everything is so interrelated that, again, the only way around this is to go to an expert in restorative medicine.

Other reasons why the thyroid may become low or underactive are because of exposure to certain viruses, a genetic inheritance, iodine deficiency, environmental toxins, autoimmune diseases or direct or indirect trauma to the thyroid gland.
Untreated, thyroid disease has been linked to chronic fatigue,

fibromyalgia, congestive heart failure, ankylosing spondylitis (a disease where the spine becomes fused, therefore suppressing movement – not very pleasant, at all), elevated cholesterol levels, heart disease, insulin resistance, muscle weakness, decreased mental function and the increased risk of cancer. Thyroid increases the number of natural killer (NK) cells which help protect against cancer. NK cells seek out and destroy cancerous cells, bombarding them with toxic enzymes. Also, we see weight gain, which is a classic symptom of hypothyroidism, and it is not uncommon for women to suffer from depression. Something that may explain this is that T3, the most active form of thyroid hormone, is also a neurotransmitter and regulates the action of serotonin, noradrenaline and GABA (gamma aminobutyric acid), which are all important brain chemicals for alleviating depression. The neurotransmitter cascade may suffer disturbances if we don't have enough T3 or it is blocked, and this may lead to mood and energy changes, including depression.

Other symptoms of low thyroid include intolerance to cold, lateral eyebrow thinning, the fatigue that I had, constipation that I also had, memory loss (cognitive dysfunction), dry and rough skin, thinning hair, being too tired to exercise (that was me), lowered body temperature, fluid retention, swollen eyelids and ankles, obesity and difficulty in losing weight, anxiety, insomnia, muscle aches, hoarseness in the mornings, hypertension and brain fog. Of course there are more, but the list is too long. Oh, and yes – brittle nails are also a sign of a thyroid deficiency.

When hypothyroidism is diagnosed, both T4 and T3 should be restored; if you only replace T4 pathways, then you may still have low thyroid symptoms because of problems with the conversion of T4 to T3. In most people, when restoring both T4 and T3, it has been seen to be much more effective. Medicines like Synthroid only contain T4 and are of the synthetic form. Armour Thyroid is made up of T4, T3, T2, T1 and other substances that assist the body in converting T4 to T3 such as calcitonin and selenium – and it is natural. Armour is desiccated thyroid or thyroid extract made from pigs' thyroid glands, that are dried and made into powder, but not to worry, this is not like the horse hormones used in the synthetic HRT. Armour is bioidentical to our body's requirements.

Low thyroid levels can cause increased cortisol production, which can lead to adrenal fatigue over time. Adrenal fatigue may make it difficult to tolerate thyroid. If our adrenals are tired, limping and therefore dysfunctional, symptoms of low thyroid may continue even when the thyroid has been balanced. This is why, again, we need an expert doctor in restorative medicine. Adrenal health should always be checked out before prescribing thyroid medication, as endeavouring to correct low thyroid levels can weaken the adrenal glands even more when there is adrenal fatigue.

Let's talk a little about iodine. Iodine is a trace element and is very important to thyroid function and hormone synthesis. Every receptor in the human body uses iodine, imagine! We need trace amounts of iodine in all of our hormone receptors for our hormones to work correctly. Iodine deficiency is very common in women and can cause hypothyroidism, especially subclinical hypothyroidism. Oestrogens inhibit the absorption of iodine so, if we have an oestrogen dominance situation, iodine will not be absorbed and we will be left deficient.

Low iodine can also cause other problems such as thyroid goitre (a benign thyroid tumour), ovarian cysts, hormonal imbalances and fibrocystic breasts. Also, a lack of iodine can contribute to severely stunted physical and mental growth, mental retardation and deafness in children due to untreated congenital hypothyroidism. So, make sure your iodine levels are good to go. Nearly 72% of the world's population is deficient in iodine. Iodine can protect against breast cancer by increasing oestriol – remember this is a cancer-protective oestrogen. Iodine is also an antibacterial, antiparasitic, antiviral agent.

Hashimoto's Thyroiditis

Hashimoto's Thyroiditis is an autoimmune disease and another form of thyroid dysfunction on the low side. Autoimmune diseases happen when the body attacks itself, which results in an inflammation of the thyroid gland. I like to describe it as the thyroid eating itself. Over time it is basically destroying its own tissue. This happens because the immune system, the body's defence mechanism, produces antibodies that bombard the thyroid and, as a result, the thyroid gland cannot manufacture enough thyroid hormone due to this attack. If antibodies are elevated and there is also hypothyroidism, this is called Hashimoto's Thyroiditis. Food allergies and intolerances that are usually associated with wheat (gluten) and other grains can aggravate this condition. Naturally, and as life would have it, this condition is far more common in women than men.

Hashimoto's Thyroiditis is not easy to understand for your 'everyday doctor'. My friend had it for years and went undiagnosed because her family doctor was not testing for optimal ranges but rather normal ranges; nor was he doing the full thyroid panel. He was doing even less than half the job. Normal ranges are not considered optimal by doctors who practise restorative medicine. Without optimal levels we are at an increased risk of premature ageing and heart disease. My friend was not treated because her ranges were considered normal by her doctor, even though she had all the symptoms, which he ignored. She was fat, unhappy and very unhealthy. Once she was diagnosed, she soon got her life back. Some of the symptoms she had were sudden weight gain, joint and muscle pain, brittle nails and thinning hair, extreme fatigue and a puffy face. She always found it difficult to get warm, she was very depressed and her menstrual cycles were often irregular and sometimes very heavy. Unfortunately, there is no cure for Hashimoto's but who cares – we now have restorative medicine. We can put back into the body what is missing and regain our quality of life and love. By restoring our hormones and correcting thyroid levels to optimal, along with iodine levels, we can combat Hashimoto's Thyroiditis, and feel really good.

Hyperthyroidism is the opposite of hypothyroidism: our thyroid produces *too much* thyroid hormone. When antibodies are elevated and there is also hyperthyroidism, this is known as Grave's disease. The most common cause of hyperthyroidism is Grave's disease. Grave's disease is another autoimmune disease only this time, instead of the thyroid not producing enough thyroid hormone, it overproduces due to the destruction (or eating up) of the thyroid gland by the autoimmune process. Again, Grave's disease is more common in women than men. It can occur at any age but the standard is between thirty and forty.

Other reasons for an overproduction of thyroid hormones can be due to taking too much thyroid medication (your family doctor did not get the full panel done), a pituitary or thyroid tumour, or a nodule on the thyroid (toxic nodular goitre). Also, some medications, such as levothyroxine (T4), may cause drug interactions that result in an overproduction of thyroid. An overproduction or too much thyroid can and will damage cells, including those of the heart and other muscles, and we will be at a higher risk of osteoporosis due to bone cell damage.

Symptoms of hyperthyroidism include weight loss – it is almost impossible to gain weight as our body's metabolism is far too high and is set on overdrive. We will get excessive sweating, hair loss, muscle weakness, a racing heart, we will be fatigued by the end of the day but find it difficult to sleep, we will also get irritable and anxious, have warm, moist skin, and maybe even trembling hands, while increased bowel movement is also common. Moodiness and depression can creep in, chest pain, puffiness around the eyes and shortness of breath. A staring gaze and slightly bulging eyeballs are also signs of hyperthyroidism. Some people may require surgery if hyperthyroidism is severe, or may be given radioactive iodine in the form of a capsule which ablates thyroid function within six weeks to six months. These treatments can cause other problems and will certainly lead to hypothyroidism or low thyroid function which will need medication. At this point, as thyroid function had been ablated, we definitely need an expert doctor to get us back on track.

Although difficult to treat, Dr Dzugan has successfully treated some cases of an overactive thyroid (hyperthyroidism) with the use of bioidentical hormones, therefore avoiding the very traumatic procedure of ablation of the thyroid gland or surgery.

Insulin

Insulin is a hormone secreted by specialised cells called the beta cells of the islet of Langerhans in the pancreas, and has a profound effect on ageing. It has many functions in the body, including energy supply to the cells, maintenance and development of muscle and other lean tissue and fat, and it also plays a major role in the production of serotonin.

Low insulin levels can be due to over-exercise, eliminating carbohydrates from our diet and not eating enough. High insulin levels can be due to consuming soft drinks, yo-yo dieting, excessive alcohol consumption or caffeine intake, diet pills, low-fat diets, smoking, deficient oestradiol levels, stress, overeating, birth control pills or artificial sweeteners. Insulin is released in the presence of sugar in the bloodstream, which helps move the glucose from the blood into the cells throughout the body; glucose cannot penetrate the cells without insulin. Insulin determines if the nutrients we take in will be used for energy or stored as fat.

As for how it works, when we consume excessive amounts of sugar, or high-glycaemic foods that are quickly converted into sugar, the pancreas releases high levels of insulin to help shuttle the sugar out of the bloodstream. We do not want high insulin levels; this will eventually provoke insulin resistance, which is a precursor to type 2 diabetes. When the cells are being continually bombarded by high insulin and sugar levels, the body sets up a defence mechanism (down-regulation) that prevents the absorption of any additional sugar. The sugar that would normally be used by the muscle (energy) is stored as fat and, of course, what happens? We put on weight. Also, an overproduction of insulin leads to high blood pressure, hardening of the arteries and free radical activity, followed by accelerated ageing and the development of disease. Not a good place to be.

In addition to being the culprit behind insulin resistance, diabetes, lifestyle complications and unwanted weight gain, high insulin levels also harm our brain cells. Our brain energises itself with sugar; it needs a certain amount, but just as important as the brain fuelling itself with sugar, there is also a need to balance these sugar levels in the brain. Otherwise, things go awry. When we become insulin resistant, our body, along with our brain, is unable to correctly balance sugar levels. This prevents correct brain fuelling and promotes brain cell destruction. Insulin resistance and diabetes also promote the destruction of a major memory-enhancing neurotransmitter, acetylcholine. Think! Your brain and memory are under significant assault every single day. I don't mean to go on but – Alzheimer's! Insulin resistance also promotes amyloids, which are proteins known to cause Alzheimer's.

As insulin is part of the hormonal network, if it is not doing its job correctly all the other hormones will be affected. Insulin levels that are continually high can cause the cells of the adrenal glands to turn on an enzyme that disrupts the body's production of oestrogens, triggering a shift towards androgen production (both oestrogens and androgens are produced from DHEA). This shift in hormonal balance alters body composition and shape, and can cause an unhealthy increase in weight. Remember, we women need oestrogens in the correct balance and ratio not only for quality of life but to protects us against Alzheimer's, osteoporosis and heart disease, to name a few.

Oestrogen(s) levels that are too low can cause excess insulin. As we age and have less oestrogens, as happens in menopause, and we accumulate more body fat, insulin receptors do not function as well as they once did. At this point, the body cannot manage the distribution of glucose as well. As a response, the pancreas releases more insulin, shuttling so much sugar into the cells that the levels in the blood plummet. Guess what the result is? Low energy levels, mood swings, and it makes us crazy for sweet foods and carbohydrates. The body is trying to bring the blood sugar up sharply. Cravings are real, they are physical. I always thought they were all in my mind (which they are in reality) when I was scouring the cupboard for bars (plural) of chocolate. Cravings are stronger than us. It is our hormones guiding us once again. Let me explain. Oestrogen(s) is one of the hormones needed to manufacture serotonin – if you remember serotonin is the 'keeps-me-happy' brain neurotransmitter. Low oestrogens make it almost impossible for a woman not to crave carbohydrates, due to the connection between oestrogens and serotonin. Low oestrogen(s) levels bring low serotonin levels. Now our brain needs a dopamine fix. Dopamine is the reward neurotransmitter, or 'God, I feel good now I have rewarded myself with that chocolate.' Now the fight really begins. Insulin levels shoot up and we need, want even more sugary stuff. The spinning top goes round and round. Low oestrogens, cravings, sugar, high glucose, insulin resistance, fat and even fatter – type 2 diabetes.

Hormonal balance is the key that protects us against a high tide of insulin in the body. A healthy diet and exercise which help reduce insulin response are also a part of this regime, but hormonal balance is bedrock to protection. We need to respect our bodies: eating healthily and exercising regularly shows respect. A body that is in perfect balance will stand firm, strong and straight. If you work well for it, it will work well for you.

OK, so what if you have a genetic predisposition? Good question. Genes are pretty impressive things. They determine the colour of our eyes, hair and many other things that give us our own distinctive looks which are inherited from our parents. They also control how cells function and how and when these functions are to be carried out. The thing is, we can control many of these genes just by the way we choose to live – managing our diet to keep our blood glucose and insulin at healthful levels is key. Excess blood glucose levels cause 'not-so-nice' gene expression that may lead to excess insulin manufacture, together with inflammation that leads to an increased risk of developing diseases such as cancer, heart disease and dementia.

Just because we have a genetic predisposition, does NOT mean that the fatal switch necessarily has to be flicked. Controlling and maintaining low glucose levels helps activate the genes that control longevity and reduce disease risk.

Adrenal Fatigue or Insufficiency

Adrenal fatigue, exhaustion or insufficiency is something you definitely don't want but many, many people are walking around with it and don't even realise – they accept it as normal, and most likely don't even know what it is. Adrenal fatigue is one of the most common yet under-diagnosed syndromes in today's society. It brings with it a feeling of being 'not so well', a lack of energy, a feeling of exhaustion but not being able to sleep, and not wanting sex anymore. Who wants it when you feel this tired anyway – you're left with your sex drive at zero. There is reduced memory and concentration, indigestion, anxiety, unexplained hair loss, poor blood sugar control, infections, alternating diarrhoea and constipation, depression and low blood pressure. The 'can't cope' syndrome that I had, and the 'everything is falling in on me' sensation.

Sleep is impossible when cortisol levels are high, but a heart attack is not. When we don't sleep it makes things worse: cortisol levels rocket even further. High cortisol raises our insulin and in turn we get fat. Also, a lack of sleep can increase circulating oestrogen(s) levels, upsetting the hormonal balance even further. When we don't sleep, more hormonal imbalances will follow. The theatre is then set for the onset of degenerative diseases. When we don't sleep, sheer exhaustion sets in and we become kind of crazy. The usual scenario when we need a pick-me-up, because we are so tired, so exhausted, so going crazy, is to reach for things like coffee, sugar, soft drinks or any stimulant that temporarily make us feel better and more energetic, but the effects are short-lived and, in the long run, this technique only worsens the situation. The negative effects greatly outweigh this short-term fix! What we need is a permanent fix.

Sleepless nights and exhausted days, together with an imbalance of hormones, usually end up with a depressed you and a cortisol dominance effect (I will explain this later). The next step is to go to our conventional doctor, who has no understanding of adrenal fatigue or burnout and who casually hands out antidepressants like Paxil or Prozac. These substances do not resolve the problem and what we are now looking at is trouble for various reasons. Certainly in the UK alone, ten thousand women a year are admitted to hospital after having been poisoned by antidepressants – this figure represents a 55% increase over five years. Although some of these women were victims of self-harm, many were addicted or had taken an overdose by accident, or suffered an allergic reaction. In most cases, the women had become dependent on these antidepressants. An estimated eighteen million prescriptions are scribbled down on prescription pads by doctors each year for sleeping pills and tranquillisers alone. Makes you think, huh?

One of the primary causes of continuous physiological stress for us is our declining hormones. Perimenopausal women have low oestrogens and progesterone levels, which put the body under an incredible and continuous stress load. If we are already highly stressed and menopausal, our stress will be exacerbated because of this – we definitely will not be sleeping. When female hormones are restored and the body is working at optimum our sleep returns. How wonderful.

Adrenal insufficiency develops gradually and is due to long-term and chronic stress, which causes the adrenals to become damaged or overworked. So what causes this breakdown?

Well, many things, things like never having a moment to relax – you know the type of person? High-energy kick, always on the move, doing, doing, doing. Always wanting to achieve, always on the edge, seeking out stressful situations. The type of person who makes sure their day is full and has one hundred things to do at once, if not a thousand things, a person who cannot relax and always wants to do more. Not being able to relax and always wanting to 'do' is definitely not a good idea! Not getting enough sleep, and environmental toxins including second-hand smoke are stressors. Chronic pain, chronic inflammation, chronic infections, hormonal imbalances, birth control pills, over-exercising, poor diet and junk food. Junk food is not a good idea; think of all those excess calories and the toxins they hold. Also, a high intake of sugar and caffeine are stressors. Stress is in our everyday life – it wasn't like that in my grandmother's time, or not to the same extent. Stress comes with financial worries, raising children, high work demands, an unhappy life and choices made, a lack of confidence and caring for a sick or elderly parent. It is truly everywhere.

When our stress levels are continuously high there is little extra cortisol for us to use in our defence when we need it. We really should learn how to control our stress and use it when we do actually need it, like in life-threatening situations. Easier said than done, right?

Prolonged stress degrades our immune systems and we all know what that means: it is not a good place to be. The invader has a greater chance of 'getting you', of getting in and making us ill, cancer included! We have difficulty fighting off infections, more so viral infections, and colds and flu are more common. Chronic, long-term stress will cause adrenal exhaustion or burnout and when that happens, we are really in trouble. You are on your way to a heart attack, if you haven't already had one.

When there is a chronic stress situation, it causes the adrenals to secrete large amounts of cortisol and adrenaline but, at the same time, the production of DHEA declines. The increased cortisol and adrenaline production will remain high and then will eventually drop to a normal level. The body then tries to adapt itself to make up for the reduced production of cortisol (in order to cope with stress) and adrenaline, by way of a phenomenon called 'pregnenolone steal'. What happens then is that pregnenonlone, DHEA, progesterone, oestrogens, testosterone and aldosterone (because pregnenolone is a precursor to all these hormones) all decline in favour of cortisol. Basically, as the term suggests, pregnenolone steal is a stealing process; it is one hormone (cortisol) stealing from another (pregnenolone) to try and adjust the production of the first hormone (cortisol) but, in this instance, the normally high cortisol compensates by going even higher, which in turn reduces the production of DHEA. The body is always trying to compensate for our daily stress but, in the end, shrugs its shoulders and gives up; it can no longer secrete adequate levels of cortisol in proportion to our levels of stress. When this happens we get adrenal exhaustion and cortisol and adrenaline become so depleted that a severe imbalance of the other steroid hormones occurs.

Please note, adrenal fatigue is not Addison's disease. With Addison's disease there is a chronic adrenal insufficiency where the adrenal glands do not produce sufficient steroid hormones (glucocorticoids and often mineralocorticoids) but, with adrenal fatigue, cortisol levels are so low that it prevents optimal functioning of the body. Adrenal fatigue is often missed or ignored by conventional doctors because they are not looking for it, or more than likely they don't even know what it is, and also because blood tests are designed to detect severe deficiency of the adrenal hormones associated with Addison's disease.

Cortisol

So, let's go on to cortisol, the 'stress hormone'. Cortisol production increases in response to any stress in the body. It is the body's survival mechanism (therefore it is healthy), and pours when the fight-or-flight response is engaged. This adaptation then quickly returns to a resting state when the stressful situation is resolved. As I stated earlier, cortisol is made in the adrenal glands. The adrenal glands do not secrete hormones at a consistent level throughout the day; in other words they fluctuate. Cortisol output is normally highest in the morning, then throughout the day it has a mid-value and at night the output drops off significantly. If a person works night shifts or sleeps at different times of the day, this pattern may change.

Unfortunately, there is a huge misconception around cortisol. Most medical doctors, including some of the most prominent, believe that cortisol levels rise with age. I also believed this to be true until Dr Dzugan explained that this was not the case, "Cortisol absolutely does not increase with age, Jill! It is a misconception!" There are many studies showing that cortisol production remains either stable or declines with age. One study conducted in 2005 by the Life Extension Foundation, and based on the data of 246 men and women aged nineteen to ninety-three, showed that cortisol levels declined with age and that the majority of patients possessed less than optimal levels of cortisol. An optimal level was found in only 28.04% of patients, and 17.88% had a cortisol level on the low side. On the other hand, only 7.72% actually had elevated cortisol levels.

A key factor of the neuroendocrine system that controls our resistance to stress is the hypothalamic-pituitary-adrenal (HPA) axis. When it breaks down, we break down! If you remember, the HPA axis is governed by the secretion of corticotropin-releasing hormone (CRH) from the hypothalamus. Once released CRH goes on to tell the pituitary gland to secrete a specific amount of adrenocorticotropic hormone (ACTH). This is a wake-up call for the adrenal glands, which then go on to determine how much cortisol is needed. If cortisol levels are high the secretion of ACTH and CRH are inhibited by way of a negative feedback loop. We will then get a breakdown.

I stated previously that there was a special relationship between DHEA and cortisol. This relationship involves the ratios between the two, known as the cortisol-to-DHEA ratio. Cortisol-to-DHEA ratio decreases when we are calm, but increases when we are under acute stress. Just as oestrogens and progesterone have a said ratio, so do cortisol and DHEA. When the cortisol-to-DHEA ratio is high we get cortisol dominance. Just as we can get oestrogen dominance, we can also get cortisol dominance. Remember the pregnenolone steal phenomenon?

When there is long-term stress our cortisol levels will remain high, which will eventually cause our adrenal glands to become damaged or exhausted. This will then cause impaired cortisol secretion and regulation. In turn, this will certainly create an imbalance between the two said ratios, which may cause high, low or normal levels of cortisol. Also, remember when the adrenal glands are exhausted we cannot maintain the proper balance of all the other steroid hormones (pregnenolone, DHEA, progesterone etc.) – stress blunts our hormone production.

Cortisol is an essential hormone for maintaining optimal health, but impaired secretion and regulation of this hormone can have devastating effects on our body. What I am saying is that prolonged, chronically elevated levels of cortisol (cortisol dominance) can be dangerous, but low levels of this hormone can be just as detrimental to our health. DHEA has a complimentary yet opposite relationship with cortisol. Something like our partners, oestrogens and progesterone. Again, it is all to do with balance. DHEA has an anabolic or building effect, whereas cortisol has a catabolic or tearing-down influence on the body. The building-up and tearing-down effects are both essential for the body; the levels and ratios of both these hormones need to be correctly balanced to counteract each other and achieve optimal health.

The consequences of a sub-par adrenal stress index (this simply refers to the ratios between these two steroid hormones, cortisol and DHEA) include osteoporosis, premature ageing, depression, insomnia, fatigue, decreased immune function and insulin resistance. Additionally, blood pressure can increase, along with cholesterol.

Thyroid problems may occur due to adrenal maladaptation. The thyroid gland directly affects adrenal hormones and assists with the conversion of thyroid hormones to the active form. The thyroid hormone (T4) that is produced may become stored and therefore unavailable for the body to use. Quite often low thyroid or symptoms of hypothyroidism such as low body temperature and fatigue are due to abnormal adrenal function.

A sub-par adrenal stress index even gets to our brain cells. Bluntly put, impaired cortisol secretion and regulation ages the brain. High levels of cortisol or cortisol dominance impairs cognitive function and can affect the way we think. It impacts on our memory, our learning abilities, our creativity. We may have more difficulty in solving problems, our reaction time may be slower, we may become forgetful and have difficulty in making decisions, we may have more difficulty in recalling and retrieving information, and we may, like me, even lose our sense of humour. Our brain is one of the body parts most affected by stress: when cortisol levels are high, or we have cortisol dominance, our body produces more free radicals, which damage the neurons affecting our ability to think and remember things. Additionally, cortisol dominance is correlated to a deterioration of the hippocampus, which is the part of the brain that processes memory. Also, elevated cortisol levels may directly contribute to Alzheimer's disease.

Cortisol works in tandem with insulin from the pancreas, making sure glucose gets to the cells where it can be burned for energy. Cortisol makes sure adequate levels of glucose are in the blood, while insulin, being the platinum key, unlocks the cell membranes to get glucose into the cells. Our body relies on glucose as the most consistent form of energy. When there is abnormal adrenal function it may alter the ability of the cells to produce the energy we need for the activities of everyday living. If you have difficulty getting up in the morning or if you have low energy levels during the day, this may be due to abnormal adrenal rhythms and poor blood sugar regulation.

When there is stress-induced cortisol secretion, we get a high cortisol to low DHEA level. Cortisol dominance can be connected to increased central body fat and can create insulin resistance. Long-term insulin resistance can cause type 2 diabetes. If insulin resistance is left unchecked it can lead to metabolic syndrome, or Syndrome X; if this condition develops, the sugar that would normally be used for energy is stored as fat instead – this is when we start to see an increase in weight. It is characterised by weight gain, especially around the abdomen – women get thicker around the stomach, waist and thighs, and men become 'potbellied'. Interestingly, when DHEA is administered (or supplemented), it has been seen to reduce the accumulation of central or abdominal visceral fat and protect against insulin resistance.

Another example of sub-par adrenal stress index is the association with depression. In an adult population a high cortisol to DHEA ratio has been linked to unipolar depression, and in adolescents a high cortisol to DHEA ratio was predictive to persistent major depression prior to the onset of unipolar depression. Also, a high morning cortisol to DHEA ratio in older men has been associated with negative mood, high anxiety and less than optimal cognitive function. Also, mood disorders such as depression and cognitive deficits, both of which characterise severe mood disorders, have been associated with elevated cortisol.

As you most likely already know, our skin regenerates mainly during the night. If you want to achieve optimal skin health, it is essential to have normal cortisol rhythms. When we have higher night cortisol values, we will get less skin regeneration. Cortisol-to-DHEA ratio needs to be balanced. Sleep is so important. Remember, poor quality of sleep, or sleep deprivation, effects the endocrine system. If we don't sleep our hormones get mixed up, and if we have an imbalance we cannot sleep. Whose tail are we chasing? Low morning cortisol and elevated evening cortisol have been associated with insomnia. We need balance.

Correct cortisol regulation is utmost to maintaining blood pressure and cardiovascular function. The words 'cortisol dominance' and 'heart attack' go hand in hand: chronically high cortisol levels lead to hypertension and nearly always to heart disease, heart attack and stroke.

When the cortisol ratio is balanced to that of DHEA, it's an incredible hormone and does some amazing things for us. It boosts our energy levels, helps ease movement in the joints, improves digestion, enhances the immune system, helps ease inflammation and pain, and stimulates appetite. It stimulates the heart, brain and circulatory and respiratory systems. Wow, quite a hormone, really. Also, with normalised cortisol levels, reverse T3 is lowered. Remember, everything is interrelated.

As you will have understood, adrenal fatigue is a symptom that greatly affects our health, but luckily can be reversed if we take the correct steps; doing things such as changing our lifestyle, eating healthily and taking dietary supplements can all help. Dr Dzugan believes that relaxation techniques may help reduce stress; techniques such as yoga, curling up with a good book, taking a hot bath, making time for sleep (although it is almost impossible to sleep with burnout, which brings with it an imbalance of hormones which worsens the situation – now we are in a vicious cycle setup), meditation, massage and exercise, but he firmly believes that stress control on a permanent basis is impossible unless and until hormonal balance is restored. With balanced hormones we regain our sleep (bliss, sheer bliss) and our balance. Without quality sleep we cannot possibly begin to think that we can restore our body to optimum; there is no way that our healing hormones have a chance to regenerate and heal without enough sleep. We have to balance our hormones to acquire quality sleep.

It can take about six months or more of continual stress for adrenal insufficiency to take hold. Once you start treatment for exhausted adrenals it can take one to two years for the glands to heal completely.

Vitamin D3

We cannot talk about steroid hormones without talking about vitamin D3. This is extremely important to health and everyone should consider taking this supplement if there is a deficiency.

Vitamin D3 is not actually a vitamin but a hormone, a secosteroid neurohormone, and functions like all steroids by turning genes on and off – this is one of the reasons why it is so critical to our health.

The reason it got called a vitamin is because it got the wrong label stuck on it, in times gone by. Vitamins are usually procured from sources outside the body, such as foods. Although some vitamin D3 is obtained through a few foods, most of it is delivered by way of direct sunlight. Again, the human body is incredible. The body is capable of manufacturing vitamin D3 simply through exposure to sunlight. Lying in the sun, in your bikini (without sunscreen on), for about twenty minutes each side, when the sun is high (10am to 3pm) should be enough to provide Vitamin D3 synthesis for most people. Long hours on the beach are really not necessary. Nearly everyone is deficient in vitamin D3, even those living in warmer climates. I certainly was. I now supplement with vitamin D3. Make sure to get your levels tested; you definitely don't want to be missing this one either.

Vitamin D3 is a product of cholesterol, and the mechanism behind it is interesting. When sunlight (UV rays) hits the skin, it converts a substance in the skin called 7-dehydrocholesterol into vitamin D3, through a series of actions. Let me explain more clearly: sun hits the skin, 7-dehydrocholesterol is produced, which then converts into that infamous substance called cholesterol, which in turn manufactures vitamin D3. Since cholesterol is a precursor to vitamin D3, we need it – cholesterol, that is. The body also needs vitamin D3 for many, many important health reasons. Vitamin D3 is turned into the prehormone 25-hydroxyvitamin D when it passes through the liver, and then into the active form when the kidneys take over. The active form is called calcitriol, or vitamin D3. Vitamin D3 synthesis declines with age mainly because the concentration of 7-dehydrocholesterol in the skin declines. It is only logical then that cholesterol-lowering drugs such as statins, or HMG CoA reductase inhibitors, which are designed to inhibit the synthesis of 7-dehydrocholesterol, also inhibit the synthesis of vitamin D3.

Vitamin D3 plays a myriad of important roles in our body. The best known is its role in calcium metabolism and bone health. Vitamin D3 facilitates the absorption of calcium from the small intestine; if there is insufficient vitamin D3, calcium will not be integrated into the bones. We have to have enough vitamin D3 for calcium to do its job, otherwise the bones will become soft; this is where the association with osteoporosis and hip fractures comes in. Taking calcium without sufficient vitamin D3 may actually weaken the bones over time.

Deficient vitamin D3 levels have been linked to practically every age-related disorder in the body, including cancer, chronic inflammation, Alzheimer's and vascular disease. Vitamin D3 has receptors throughout the body, especially in the brain, helping to protect us against Alzheimer's.

Without sufficient vitamin D3 levels we cannot expect to be healthy and stay healthy. Vitamin D3 is vital for our body and its defence mechanism, the immune system. Remember, there is no way we can be healthy if our immune system is down. Also, vitamin D3 affects at least two hundred genes, some of which regulate cancer cell growth and differentiation, protecting us against cancers such as breast, colon, skin and prostate. These genes also regulate cell death and limit the growth of tumour blood supplies.

When vitamin D3 levels are optimal, we have a significantly reduced risk of developing many cancers, including the above mentioned along with ovary, cervix, oesophagus, pancreas, uterus, rectum, bladder, lung and kidney. Please remember that vitamin D3 levels must be optimal and not just normal to reap these benefits. It is important to get them checked by a doctor practising restorative medicine. It is only sensible to protect ourselves and supplement with vitamin D3, if there is a deficiency, to prevent health problems that could occur later in life.

6. LIFETIME TRANSITIONS

Now we have discussed the minor and major hormones, let's go over what happens to our body and its lifetime transitions.

Isn't life wonderful until we hit midlife? Well, almost wonderful! We transition from childhood into puberty, with all its discomforts and madness. Hormone levels are fluctuating all over the place, which brings with it confusion and lack of understanding and tolerance toward life and our parents. Do you remember that? I always thought my parents were being difficult but in reality it was my hormones playing dirty on me, a hormonal revolt. I was all mixed up and could not say I felt happy. I hated my body and thought I was fat when in reality it was my body making the transition from childhood into womanhood. Oestrogens were never that good to me, I never became really curvaceous or sexy; rather, I had a slight frame but with a well-rounded, full bottom (butt) and an average-size bust.

I remember I was thirteen when I had my first period. It was the day after my birthday, so I was just out of being twelve. So young. My breasts hurt and I had what they called a lump – no breast at all, really. I had one pubic hair and no hair under my arms. Incredible. I didn't even know what a period was. I went to the bathroom and found blood. I ran downstairs screaming, thinking I was going to die. That's how ignorant I was about life. My mother had never told me. I suppose she didn't expect me to start so early. Luckily my friend, Christine Pye, was there. Her mother was a nurse. It was the school holidays and the only one around, apart from my friend, was my grandfather and I surely didn't feel like telling him. Christine explained to me that it was a normal process, and that I was not dying. I had become a woman. She took me down to her mother's, who gave me a huge sanitary towel,

Dr White's – do you remember those terrible things? I told my mother that evening and she took it in her stride, saying, "Well, you are a woman now, Jill, but so early!" I hated the fact that I had to have periods and many of my friends didn't. It was so embarrassing for me, especially when I was obliged to sit out of the gym or sports class.

It took a while for my periods to become regular, my hormones, along with madness and mood swings, fluctuating all the time. Once that transition passed and my periods were regular I felt good, normal again. I was reproductive and feeling positive. From about the age of sweet sixteen to forty-six I had very regular, almost to the second, periods. The only problem I had as an adult woman was carrying my pregnancies to full term. I realise now how lucky I was getting such regular periods – it was a sign I was hormonally balanced.

From about age twenty to thirty we are at our peak; our body is at its best (although I never had a good relationship with my body – it was all psychological, of course, I was fine really), firm and strong, with clear thinking, over-the-top energy, positivity and an attitude that leads us to think we can do and get anything we want. We are well on our way to building our adult future.

Then we hit the mid-forties and fifties, or sometimes earlier, and there is another transition, just when we'd been feeling so good. It had to happen! Could it be that we've entered perimenopause, the precursor to the dreaded menopause? Oh no, not possible! Women today are entering perimenopause earlier due to stress and toxicity. Perimenopause usually happens five to ten years prior to menopause, and highlights a decline in and fluctuation of ovarian oestrogens, along with progesterone. What happens is, as oestrogens decline, there is an increase in a hormone called FSH (follicle-stimulating hormone). FSH stimulates ovarian oestrogen(s) production but when there is a decline, the production of FSH increases to try and restore oestrogen(s) production, with no luck. A fully reproductive woman will make sufficient oestrogens to create a peak on the twelfth day to continue the monthly cycle.

Oestrogen and Progesterone Levels During a 28-Day Menstrual Cycle

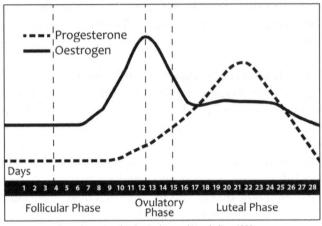

Source: *Principles and Practice of Endocrinology and Metabolism*, 1990

Without this peak the message cannot be relayed so the release of any of the eggs we have left does not occur. Without this feedback information we cannot shut off FSH. So, FSH continues to flow constantly and, because of this mechanism, it over-stimulates the ovaries and triggers the eradication of the rest of the eggs we have left. Excess FSH uses up the remainder of our eggs and that, my dear friend, is the system effectively shutting itself down for the rest of our days. Hey-ho, we are in full-blown menopause.

Perimenopause brings with it another shift in our hormones, only this time, unlike puberty, our hormones are in decline; it's puberty in reverse. In puberty our hormones are getting ready to build us up for better things to come, for reproduction, an adult future, full of energy, power and sharp thinking. Although we are at different stages in our lives, hormones are hormones and the emotional feelings will be the same both in puberty and perimenopause. We will cry more easily, be less tolerant and understanding, anger will get the better of us when it shouldn't, we will get teen rages, an illogical hit of pure negative energy. We will even get depressed. You may get the 'no one understands me' feeling and the 'can't cope' syndrome, you may feel used and abused and unappreciated. I got all of that, when in actual fact, it was not true; no more so than it had ever been. It was a hormonal imbalance called perimenopause. Hormones are pretty crazy things. They rule us.

In perimenopause the machine is running on nearly empty; that is why we just don't feel right. In perimenopause we have almost no eggs left, so that means we don't have many oestrogens left either. That's why our periods may become erratic, they may become lighter or heavier than usual, or we may get bleeding in between them. We may get painful, lumpy breasts that get lumpier and lumpier, and we are at greater risk of breast cancer. This is the age where the balance between oestrogens and progesterone will shift heftily toward oestrogens, creating an oestrogen dominance effect. And, of course, we will not want sex anymore. How depressing. How could this have happened? Sex had always been instinctive, natural, good.

The path is laid out, and it is one we are destined to follow. Full-blown menopause is on its way. But we are luckier now and can miss that part out if we want to and just age gracefully, happily and healthily, with none of the traditional ailments and age-related diseases due to severe hormonal loss. We do not have to follow the old template of ageing and conventional medical care. We have a choice; why not take it? Why suffer the discomforts and dangers of the menopause and ageing when there is a new approach, encompassed with knowledge and power, a knowledge that includes clarity, efficiency and safety? We can enjoy this transition, this change of life, and be secure in our health and safety. We have emerging science and powerful doctors on our doorstep, and they have come to us to offer us the best in health. Restore your hormones and enjoy the second half of your life instead of fearing it.

Menopause means the end of our reproductive life. We have no eggs left and without eggs there will be no oestrogen(s) production and consequently this leads to no more progesterone production either. The brain does not like this scenario; it likes to think we are still reproductive. Yes, it may sound crazy but it's true. It gets confused and thinks we are of no use anymore. It believes we are only there to reproduce. Yes, you may say, a brain that is not so clever after all. But it is. It is reading exactly what the body is giving it, or not giving it. Biologically speaking we are here to perpetuate the species. If we restore these missing hormones with bioidentical ones we are resetting the brain into thinking all is well – life will go on as before, even if we are no longer capable of making babies. Remember, hormones regenerate and regulate, they are the essence of life itself. Restoring our hormones helps us to avoid age-related diseases and the cancer that is in all of us. We all have cancer in us. A woman in her fifties is at greater risk of contracting breast cancer because of the initial hormonal imbalances she went through in perimenopause. This is the time when the cancer she already has in her body, that is lying dormant and peaceful, has a chance to proliferate and grow. This is a major reason perimenopause should be, has to be, taken seriously. Tell your friends, tell your doctors. Balance is everything. When we have balance we have health. Without it… do I need to repeat myself?

7. MENOPAUSAL BREAKDOWN OF THE BODY

Let's talk about some of the things menopause brings with it. We'll start with the most superficial of things, the skin. But, remember, the skin is giving us the first signs of body breakdown. It is talking to us, letting us know what is happening inside our body, that we are ageing. If we are ageing on the outside then we are slowly but surely ageing on the inside as well.

When we hit menopause the mirror becomes our unwanted friend. We are obliged to look at it but we don't enjoy it like we used to; the sight is, well, slightly depressing. Quite suddenly and drastically after menopause our skin seems to shrivel up and become paper-thin, wrinkles deepen and become more apparent. Elasticity – well, there's no stretch anymore. The skin becomes drier and we bruise more easily and heal less quickly. These changes in the skin are partly due to a decline in oestrogen(s) levels; a constant reminder of our fading youth.

Well, not for me, I'm not having it. A decline in oestrogens creates a loss of collagen, hyaluronic acid and other significant substances. When I look at the skin of my youngest son's girlfriend, who is seventeen, and see how puffy and full and youthful her skin is I realise how lucky I was – at the time I didn't think about it. Young skin's beauty, elasticity and glow are there because of youthful levels of collagen, which is a protein that assists not only skin but bone, tendons and cartilage, helping to give them their quality and strength. Women start losing collagen in their early forties, which coincides with the early days of perimenopause and a decline in oestrogens. Around the same time there is also a slowing-down of new skin cell formation and the dying off of the old ones. Old cells seem to want to hang on, causing the skin to become dull, thick and wrinkly.

Balanced oestrogen(s) levels help keep skin from ageing so drastically. By simply replacing with bioidentical oestrogens (and, of course, remember, never to use oestrogens exclusively; we always have to balance with progesterone) when there is a decline we can maintain and even erase some of the years of ageing skin. Although oestrogen(s) levels have always been connected with skin maintenance, it was never quite sure how. Now we know. Skin cells are covered with oestrogen(s) receptors so when oestrogens bind to these receptors the structure of elastic fibres is improved. Also, it encourages the growth of new blood vessels in the skin, which helps control the inflow of nutrients and the outflow of waste. Bioidentical oestrogens increase skin thickness and water content by stimulating the growth of particular cells called fibroblasts and keratinocytes, and by promoting the release of substances including mucopolysaccharides and hyaluronic acid. Of course, this is just part of the story about skin health – testosterone, progesterone, DHEA and growth hormone also contribute towards a younger-looking skin.

A Beauty Hint – My Little Secret

Let me tell you a little secret, ladies. There are lots of little things we can do to improve the quality of our skin. One little trick of mine is to use (E3) oestriol cream, topically compounded with antioxidants. This natural mix gives amazing results. My skin, I would say over a period of two to three months, became thicker and showed an increase in moisture; I was literally glowing. Elasticity and firmness improved, my shallow wrinkles became even less apparent and pore size decreased. Not bad for a fifty-four-year-old – I feel good! You need a prescription for this; you cannot just go out and buy it. Avoid buying petroleum-based products if you want a younger-looking skin.

Like I said, skin shows us the first signs of ageing and many hormonal imbalances can be reflected in it. Acne may appear if testosterone is too high or, if testosterone is too low, we may get saggy skin. If there is an imbalance we may get rosacea, which is an inflammatory skin condition. Your skin tells the truth. You can have beautiful skin even at fifty and sixty and maybe beyond. Balance your hormones.

Weight Gain

Unexpected weight gain is very common in perimenopause. All my friends have increased their body weight since entering menopause. I, on the other hand have not, nor have I become square round the middle. I am on bioidentical hormones. I have restored my body and, boy oh boy, am I happy – muscular and thin, but still feminine. I have maintained my weight and body shape since age twenty-six. I know I would have gained weight had I not embraced restorative medicine. I was definitely on the way there. I could have dieted and exercised all I liked but the weight would have gone on anyway. My body had become sluggish; it was the beginnings of menopause that was to blame. A decline in hormonal production slows us down and is biologically problematic.

One of the reasons we gain weight in perimenopause is because there is an imbalance of hormones. The hormonal environment is usually one of high insulin, along with low oestrogens and thyroid function. When our minor hormones decline, as they do during menopause, our majors rise – it's a feedback mechanism, our body is trying to right itself. We cannot lose weight if we have high insulin or if our thyroid is dysfunctional. My thyroid was low; that's one of the reasons I found it hard to get up in the morning, to get started. I had become lethargic. When we have low thyroid it doesn't matter how much we diet or exercise, the weight will NOT come off. Our body cannot metabolise the food we eat effectively, turning calories into fat instead of using them for energy.

When female hormones are low it puts an enormous stress on the body. If you remember, stress causes cortisol to rise. When cortisol levels are high, we store more fat, because cortisol facilitates the storage of fat. High cortisol or cortisol dominance also increases the breakdown of muscle and insulin resistance. When cortisol levels continue to be high or dominant the body goes into 'flight or fight' mode, which instigates weight gain. We need balance.

The ratio of ovarian hormones usually decides how much weight we put on and in which area of the body we retain it. If, let's say, the ratio of oestradiol (E2) is high to progesterone, weight gain may be around the hips. But if oestradiol decreases and progesterone is normal, along with testosterone and DHEA, then we will most likely put weight on around the middle. Women with balanced hormones are less likely to gain weight than those without. Balance your hormones.

Note: Excess body fat holds excess oestrogens. Fat cells contain an enzyme (aromatase) that converts testosterone into E2 (oestradiol), and this is the reason why overweight and obese women have more oestradiol. After menopause oestrogens are mostly produced in body fat, that is, in the buttocks, thighs and breasts. When a woman is overweight her breast tissue will be fatty, leading to higher levels of oestrogens in the breast. Overweight and obese women have more oestrogens, and the more oestrogens produced in the breast, the more likely it is to give way to the growth of breast cancer cells.

The Brain Change and Misty Thinking!

The brain change and misty thinking in perimenopause is largely due to the decline in oestrogens, although a balance of other key hormones is also required for clear thinking. Pregnenolone is considered a powerful hormone for maintaining healthy cognitive function. It is the first hormone to be produced from cholesterol and generates a host of key neurohormones in the brain. Ensuring optimal levels of pregnenolone enhances memory, reduces the risk of dementia and alleviates anxiety and depression.

Let's also take a look at our female hormones, oestrogens, and how they affect the brain. Oestrogens protect the brain in many ways: without optimal oestrogen(s) levels our thinking power will slow, retrieval time for facts will be less quick and our memory will definitely decline. I lost my car, remember? We *will* develop senior moments, those terribly embarrassing moments when you can't remember his or her name, or when the project you've just been working on that you have to talk about suddenly seems insurmountable because you can't remember half the words you need to say – not good when you need a high degree of intellectual control. It doesn't make you look good. It affects your everyday life, and your career may depend on it. This is what happens in perimenopause; it is a normal process, but does not have to be – our hormones become imbalanced and our brain is rewiring.

Who wants to lose their thinking power at forty or fifty? It would be sad to have to let go of this experienced, efficient and sophisticated, yet more mature, brain. You don't have to. Our brain moves from naiveté to wisdom because of the experiences we gain throughout life. We mature, we know where we are going. This is something I lost but got back – clarity; sharp, power-thinking. With all the experiences I have acquired throughout life, my brain is now at its best. I have restored my body and by doing so I have restored my brain. I will not let go of that. As I stated earlier, female hormones are extremely potent modulators of the brain chemicals serotonin, GABA and dopamine. When oestrogen(s) levels drop, so do serotonin (the feel-good neurotransmitter) levels. In fact, when there is a rapid change in oestrogen(s) levels and serotonin levels decline, it can cause depression. Oestrogens also increase the production of a certain neurotransmitter called acetylcholine, which is required for optimal brain function (memory and learning). Also, oestradiol binds to the cortex, hippocampus and the basal forebrain, which are all areas that help with memory.

And listen to this: women taking oestrogens have better verbal memory (brain-to-mouth connection – we don't forget words when we are speaking) than women who are not on oestrogens. And, just to give you another backup, women's verbal memory decreases after a hysterectomy with removal of the ovaries (oophorectomy), but returns to normal following hormone restoration. Progesterone also plays a significant role in memory – partners in crime. They stop the brain drain. Testosterone, which is the precursor to oestradiol, not only increases one's libido but is also necessary for increased cognitive functioning.

Oestrogens also decrease distractibility. Remember when I said I was always distracted in those years of hormonal revolt and bumped into the back of that car? Well, I don't do that anymore; I mean I am not distracted and I don't bump into the back of cars anymore. My brain is amazing, sharp and quick-thinking. And my memory – well. When I am researching, the information stays in there, it doesn't just float around for a few hours and out again. My brain absorbs it like a sponge and retains it. I got my memory back.

High endogenous (produced in the body) oestradiol levels are important in their connection to Alzheimer's; women with the highest endogenous levels of oestradiol have a far lower risk of contracting Alzheimer's disease. So, what's your answer? Restoration of the body.

Alzheimer's, Alzheimer's everywhere – we just can't get away from it. Alzheimer's disease is much more common in women. Restoring our oestrogen(s) levels, along with progesterone, helps protect us against Alzheimer's disease. Women like myself are half as likely to get Alzheimer's disease as women who are not on oestrogens. And time is of essence here: the sooner the better. We need to restore our hormones before Alzheimer's has taken over and our brain has become one tangled mess. Restoring oestrogens in postmenopausal women may delay the start of Alzheimer's, but restoring when the damage is already done will do nothing. Alzheimer's cannot be reversed.

While we are on about the brain and Alzheimer's, let's talk about excitotoxins. You can see the word 'toxins' at the end of that term, so you understand it is something to do with toxicity. It is very important you understand what excitotoxins are and the role oestrogens play in protecting our brain from them.

Glutamates, aspartate and cysteine are three amino acids that excite our neurons. We have neurotransmitters that excite and neurotransmitters that calm our neurons. The above three neurotransmitters excite. When there is an overabundance of these amino acids in the brain it can cause the neurons to die. Food manufacturers are now adding these excitotoxins to the many processed foods we eat today, including baby foods. They are very dangerous brain toxins and cause damage to the nervous system. What happens when we consume these excitotoxins is that the neurons in our brain become over-excited and start firing off rapid impulses until they become totally exhausted and then suddenly die, never to be reborn. Nearly every tissue in our body has glutamate receptors and when they are over-activated by excess glutamate consumption, over time this can create a host of disorders including heart failure, atherosclerosis, diabetes, lung damage, Alzheimer's and cancer – in other words, they mess with the body. Glutamates make tumours grow at a greater rate, and make them invasive. Tumours have glutamate receptors and prognosis is dependent on the number of these glutamate receptors. Also, glutamates make chemotherapy less effective.

Glutamate is one of the most common neurotransmitters (neurotransmitters send messages by interacting with receptors). Once this neurotransmitter (glutamate) binds to the receptor, it becomes very excited. Glutamates drastically affect the neuroendocrine system, and the regulation of all our hormones is directly and profoundly affected by excess glutamates. Oestrogens are very potent inhibitors of excitotoxicity and are protective of the brain. In menopause there is a decline in oestrogens, so their role in protecting the brain is diminished. Ensure your oestrogen(s) levels are optimal, ladies. Given in physiological doses, oestrogens protect the brain. It is known that in men, when testosterone is too high or above physiological levels, it is very toxic to the brain and accentuates excitotoxicity. When bioidentical hormones are given in the correct physiological doses, it reduces the incidence of Alzheimer's disease and is very protective of the brain. You need the right amount; you need balance.

When buying processed foods, check your labels for hydrolysed protein, vegetable protein extract, autolysed yeast extract and natural flavour – these are all hidden names for MSG (Monosodium glutamate). Do not drink diet soda drinks because you will be exposing yourselves to very high amounts of aspartame that over time induce cancer. Aspartame also attacks the brain, causing brain damage similar to that caused by glutamates.

Hysterectomy

My sister had a full hysterectomy (including oophorectomy – ovaries removed as well) because of a possible cancer risk in her uterus, due to taking tamoxifen. Remember, tamoxifen inhibits in the breast but stimulates in the uterus. The trouble is that many women, when approaching menopause, have complaints related to the uterus, including abnormal bleeding. Periods may be light or sometimes heavy, or even very heavy, and haemorrhaging may occur. Periods may become irregular, arriving later or sooner than expected – these changes are all due to hormonal loss. Before the hormonal decline our periods are usually regular, but suddenly they become erratic. Why? Because our hormones are askew. Unfortunately, most women who have haemorrhaging or heavy bleeding are advised to have a full hysterectomy (with oophorectomy) to avoid cancer and are told that their ovaries will eventually stop producing hormones anyway. This is what is known as surgical menopause. Never trust a man/woman who says, "Trust me." Your doctor is not a bad man/woman, but he/she is not to be trusted. He/she is leading you down the road to doom and gloom, and a 'fast-forward' old age. These women, like my sister, soon found out that a life without hormones is not so good. A hysterectomy, with or without oophorectomy, decreases circulating levels of testosterone, which creates an imbalance.

Women who have had a partial hysterectomy (without oophorectomy) also have a change in hormonal production, which can happen over a period of three to four years after the operation. The decline occurs because the uterine artery has been cut and tied off, decreasing the blood flow to the ovaries. Surgical menopause is much more drastic than natural menopause because the body is suddenly and violently sent into menopause, and without any warning.

Breakthrough and abnormal bleeding are symptoms; our uterus is talking to us. It is telling us that there is a hormonal imbalance that needs correcting. The uterus bleeds when there is a hormonal imbalance. Taking away the uterus – the evidence, as it were – does not correct the underlying problem. There is a hormonal imbalance which will remain, even when the evidence is taken away. This will set the stage for possible cancer eruption. Bleeding is a warning that things are going wrong. Restoring with bioidentical hormones in rhythm so the oestrogen(s) receptor sites can open up to receive progesterone is what is needed at this point.

Women who have had a hysterectomy, especially those who have had their ovaries removed, will, of course, be able to have sex again, but they will definitely not be able to *feel* sex again – there is a big difference. The majority of women are never told about this before they have their female organs cut away from them. Restoring their bodies with full hormone replacement, which means taking oestrogens and progesterone in a way that mimics our natural cycle, will help with this problem. Most women are given synthetic oestrogens, which are meant to manage hot flushes, but no progesterone, and given a pat on their back and sent on their way. A sad, no-sex-life life! To make things even worse, we gain weight, depression follows and sleep disappears. Life is looking dim. In fact, very dim – their risk for heart disease, osteoporosis, macular degenerative disease, cognitive decline, diabetes and/or cancer has just shot to the sky.

The sooner bioidentical hormones are restored, the better; the benefits will be much more effective in the long run. Can you imagine a life without hormones? I certainly can't. Doom and gloom and chronic disease is what springs to mind. Hormone restorative therapy is fine-tuned and individualised; you need to restore your body so you can keep on loving and living. You don't want or need a pat on your back, you want and need to restore your body. It is your life and you're the one who has to live with it and look after it.

Fibromyalgia

Although fibromyalgia is not a condition that necessarily starts in perimenopause, it does affect a high percentage of women. In fact, 75–90% of fibromyalgia patients are women, and it can get worse in the perimenopausal phase as our hormones decline, so I felt it necessary to discuss this condition, especially since Dr Dzugan has proved that it is reversible with the use of restorative medicine. This is so exciting, and real. Conventional medicine claims that fibromyalgia is irreversible and focuses on alleviating symptoms by giving medicines such as antidepressants, non-steroidal anti-inflammatory drugs (NSAIDs), painkillers, psychoactive drugs or lidocaine injections with or without hydrocortisone, and advises the patient to do gentle stretching, moderate exercise, physical therapy, stress-reduction techniques such as meditation, and cognitive behavioural therapies (CBT). There are two specific medicines that are prescribed for fibromyalgia, called pregabalin (Lyrica) and milnacipran (Savella). Why do we need these nasty chemicals in our body, with all the side effects, including dizziness, blurred vision and weight gain, when there is a safe, more natural way, without any side effects?

It is estimated that a whopping two hundred to four hundred million people worldwide have fibromyalgia syndrome, that is 3–6% of the population. The main symptoms of fibromyalgia syndrome are characterised by widespread pain, tenderness at specific points and fatigue, and the condition is quite difficult to diagnose. It usually develops somewhere between the ages of twenty to fifty-five. People who have other rheumatic diseases, such as rheumatoid arthritis or lupus, are more likely to develop fibromyalgia. Of course, fibromyalgia is not life-threatening but it does significantly diminish quality of life. I could not imagine living with continual pain, and think about the stress it must put on our body! We will have elevated cortisol levels, or cortisol dominance.

In addition to the typical symptoms above, people with fibromyalgia may have muscle and joint stiffness when getting up from bed or after sitting for long periods of time in a certain position; facial pain, which may often be accompanied by pain in the muscles that move the jaw – this is known as temporomandibular joint dysfunction; headaches; irritable bowel syndrome; memory loss; confusion; burning or tingling in the extremities; allergies; restless leg syndrome; depression and/or anxiety; sleeping problems – and they may be hypersensitive to sound, light or odours (all these symptoms can be classified as neuroimmunoendocrinological). A lot of symptoms. Do any of you recognise these symptoms? There is now a cure. You can start living again.

As fibromyalgia is a complex condition, the medical profession has not been able to put its finger on why it happens and where it comes from – until now, at least. One theory that the conventional medical profession has suggested is that the HPA (hypothalamic-pituitary-adrenal) axis may be hyperactive or hypoactive, meaning there is no balance. Another theory is that it is caused by an irreversible disturbance of the neuroimmunoendocrinological system. Remember, if the body is to function correctly, all systems must function correctly; they are all interrelated. The brain, immune system and endocrine system have to be balanced. Dr Dzugan agrees with the neuroimmunoendocrinological theory, but does not agree with the irreversible part. *It is reversible!* He has shown that to be so.

To explain: hormonal deficiencies in people with fibromyalgia are associated with a loss of sensitivity of cell membranes to hormonal messages. Hormones are not conversing well with cells; there is a lack of communication. This will then lead to a dysfunction of the autonomic nervous system (ANS). Remember, the ANS works with the endocrine system through the hypothalamus to delegate hormonal secretions – hormones either make or break us.

Based on Dr Dzugan's clinical experience and analysis of medical literature, he has found, and his evidence definitely shows, that fibromyalgia syndrome is a combination of neuroendocrinological and metabolic disorders and hormonal balances. The fact that most people with fibromyalgia are women in their reproductive years shows a very close and transparent link between sex hormones and metabolic disorders. Also, fibromyalgia is linked to retarded menstruation and reduced fertility, both of which are signs of a hormonal imbalance. And, to go on, chronic and widespread musculoskeletal pain (which involves the entire system of muscles, tendons and ligaments, and bones and joints that move the body and keep it standing tall), fatigue, sleep problems, gastrointestinal complaints and psychological problems are symptoms of fibromyalgia and are also associated with hormonal deficiencies.

Women with fibromyalgia, more often than not, have low melatonin levels. When they supplement with this hormone it helps to reduce pain, helps with sleep disturbances and reduces depression. Chronic stress causes cortisol levels to rise, which has been seen to provoke the development of fibromyalgia. Remember, elevated cortisol levels or cortisol dominance mess with neuroendocrine function. This may explain why this happens.

The symptoms of fibromyalgia and the side effects of statin drugs are similar. Statins lower cholesterol, which will lead to a decreased production of hormones, which will in turn lead to a hormone imbalance. Remember, we need cholesterol to produce hormones; it's our manufacturing plant.

So, following on, when hormone restorative therapy was introduced to patients suffering with this condition, symptoms of fibromyalgia disappeared. What I am saying is that fibromyalgia is the result of hormonal deficiencies which cause a breakdown in neurohormonal and metabolic integrity. It's our hormones again that rule us, make or break us. They are the leaders of the pack. They are the ones that talk, instruct and balance our bodily systems. Balance is everything.

In one way, fibromyalgia is a very complex condition but, to sum it up easily, fibromyalgia is coming from 'the common denominator' i.e. a hormonal deficiency. You need to restore your body and live again. Peace… just think.

Breast Cancer

First of all, I would just like to say that most types of cancers are preventable by making *lifestyle* changes – living a *deathstyle* type of life will only lead to an early grave. As I mentioned earlier, diet and exercise are important factors for increasing or decreasing cancer risk. Exercise has a great influence on our body and how it functions, and has been shown to decrease nearly all cancers by almost 50%, while vigorous exercise decreases our risk of breast cancer by 30%. Exercise also helps reduce other risk factors for cancer such as poor diet, smoking and being overweight. Being overweight has many negative effects on our body and can increase our oestrogen(s) levels and insulin, which can increase the rate of cancer cell growth. Increased insulin tends to increase insulin-like growth factor-1 (IGF-1), both of which promote the growth of breast cancer. Also, in overweight women, the risks of getting endometrial and gall bladder cancer are five times higher.

Back to diet. Eating a low glycaemic index diet is more protective against breast cancer, as opposed to eating a high glycaemic index diet. Eating a high glycaemic diet, along with too much red meat, may increase our risk of developing breast cancer by nearly 60%. And, incredibly, over 90% of breast tumours are insulin-receptor positive, meaning that diets high in carbohydrates, sugars and high glycaemic foods are directly connected to the development and progression of breast cancer.

Lung cancer is the leading cause of cancer death in women, but breast cancer is the second. Women working nightshifts over an extended period of time have an increased risk of developing breast cancer. This may be due to the prolonged exposure to light, which lowers melatonin levels. Remember, melatonin is a powerful antioxidant and helps protect against cancer.

Prolonged stress, as I mentioned earlier, heightens the risk of developing any form of cancer, but this is especially so with breast cancer. Long-term stress reduces the breakdown (methylation) of oestrogens in the body. Oestrogens are not then broken down into the 'good oestrogens' (remember, we have 'good' and 'bad' oestrogens) that help decrease our risk of breast cancer. When this occurs the breakdown groups (methyl groups) that are involved in the breakdown (methylation) get used up by the body to make adrenaline. We need to avoid stress but, as I have already stated, Dr Dzugan firmly believes that stress control on a permanent basis is impossible unless and until hormonal balance is restored.

Cruciferous foods, such as cabbage, broccoli, Brussels sprouts, cauliflower, bok choy, kale, kohlrabi, rutabaga and turnips can all improve the breakdown (methylation) of oestrogens in our body and help decrease our risk of developing breast cancer. We spoke about the three oestrogens, oestradiol, oestrone and oestriol, earlier on. Oestradiol and oestrone can be converted into each other, which helps to keep these hormone levels balanced. Now let's just take this one step further. Oestradiol that does not get converted into oestrone has three possible options thereafter: oestriol (which cannot be converted back), 2-hydroxyestradiol or 16a-hyrdoxyestradiol. Some of the 2-hydroxyestradiol can be turned into a metabolite called 2-methoxyestrone.

Now, looking at oestrone. Oestrone that does not get converted into oestradiol has two possible options thereafter: 2-hydroxyestrone or 16a-hydroxyestrone and, following on, some 2-hydroxyestrone can be converted into 2-methoxyestrone, and some 16a-hydroxyestrone can be changed into oestriol. Remember, oestriol is a by-product of oestradiol and oestrone.

It is vitally important that you understand that there are good and bad oestrogens all the way down the line, which may have an influence on breast cancer risk.

The 2/16 Ratio

So, to continue, 2-hydroxyestrone is considered a 'good' oestrogen metabolite, while 16a-hydroxyestrone is considered a 'bad' oestrogen metabolite. 2-hydroxyestrone is a weak but 'good' oestrogen, and non-carcinogenic and may even be anti-carcinogenic, whereas 16a-hydroxyestrone is a more powerful but 'bad' oestrogen, more potent than oestradiol and extremely toxic to our DNA. This is known as the 2/16 ratio. Anything that upsets the balance of this ratio (good to bad oestrogens) could increase the risk of oestrogen(s)-related cancers. So, if 2-hydroxyestrone (good) levels are higher than 16a-hyrdoxyestrone (bad) levels, our risk of developing breast cancer (along with uterus, prostate in men, liver and kidney cancers) may be increased. Optimal levels are considered to be twice as much 'good' oestrogen to 'bad' oestrogen, a 2:1 ratio, in other words.

The supplement known as indole 3-carbinol (I3C) is rich in a variety of phytochemicals, some with anti-cancer activity, that are found in cruciferous vegetables. I take one every day.

Indole 3-carbinol boosts levels of 2-hyrdoxyestrone, the good metabolite, and squelches the manufacture of the potent, bad, carcinogenic metabolite 16a-hydroxyestrone. Indole 3-carbinol increases the 2/16 ratio. We need the 2 to be higher for better protection against breast cancer.

Hot Flushes and Night Sweats

Hot flushes and night sweats are probably one of the most common menopausal symptoms. They are transitional and last only as long as it takes our hormones to adapt. Nevertheless, they are very, very annoying and happen at the times when we least want them to happen. This is the beginning of the end, unless you restore your body.

Why and how do hot flushes happen? Inhibin is a hormone produced by the ovaries. In perimenopause this hormone declines and, as a result, a message is received by the pituitary gland (in the brain – we are communicating again) that a diminished amount is being produced. To try and compensate for this loss, the pituitary gland then releases FSH (follicle-stimulating hormone), in an attempt to provoke (stimulate) the ovaries to produce more inhibin. This increase brings with it an increased production of all other ovarian hormones, primarily oestrogens. The continual decline in this hormone will create a continual higher production of FSH. It is this loss of inhibin that creates the initial symptoms of hot flushes and night sweats. Because of this mechanism we have an increased production in oestrogens by the ovaries, which will cause symptoms of excess oestrogens or oestrogen dominance (breast swelling, bloating and bleeding), even though we are having hot flushes. It is inhibin that initially triggers hot flushes in perimenopause.

Eventually inhibin will fall to zero, and when this happens, inhibin is no longer able to control FSH production. We are left with an increased production of FSH and an excessive increase in the production of oestrogens. The best way to correct this is to restore and balance your body.

Sexual Happiness

The majority of women at this stage of their lives will be disinterested in sex. This is because our sex hormones are declining; we are entering perimenopause, and menopause and post-menopause don't get any better. It's a common event, even if some women don't like to admit it. It is also very unfair, especially if you are married to a man more or less the same age as you. He will most likely want it all the time; you, on the other hand, may feel depressed, persistently fatigued and generally unwell. And sex, well, it hurts anyway; it is uncomfortable.

For the first thirty-five to forty years of our lives, before 'the decline', oestrogens are primarily produced in the ovaries, and rhythmically flow through our body along with progesterone and testosterone, keeping it healthy and in balance, while we are reproductive and having a great time sexually. Our curiosity and need for sex begins in adolescence when our hormones are building us up for a better future. The link is our sex hormones; it is when these hormones decline that our sexuality fades. Both oestrogens and progesterone are needed to maintain women's sexual organs in a normal and healthy condition. Testosterone is needed for sexual desire, arousal and fantasy. In menopause, things start going wrong – 'the decline'. Ovarian oestrogens have many functions, one of which is to aid our sexual happiness. It supports the blood flow to the vaginal lining but, with a decline of this hormone, the blood flow to the genital area becomes lesser, which causes genital tissue to lose its sensitivity, leading to reduced arousal and greater difficulty in achieving orgasm. Also, vaginal tissue tends to become dryer and thinner, leaving the vaginal walls more susceptible to infection and irritation, making sexual intercourse painful and uncomfortable. It is important to restore your body if you want to enjoy sex again, although admittedly, it is not all to do with sex but let's face it, you won't want sex if you are not healthy. And, if you don't restore your body, you cannot be healthy – it's all interconnected. Vaginal dryness and atrophy are commonplace in menopausal women.

Balance your body and you will avoid these problems and at the same time protect yourself from illness and age-related diseases.

Leaky Bladder Syndrome

Another common symptom of menopause is 'leaky bladder' and pain or difficulty in urinating – I had that too; I mean difficulty in urinating, not actually leaky bladder, which occurs more often in older women (post-menopause). Of course, I had no idea why this was happening, but now I know. Something was missing. This syndrome is due to a weakened muscle in the bladder and urethra (the tube that releases urine out of the body). The overall health and strength of these muscles is largely dependent on balanced oestrogen(s) levels; when there is a low oestrogen(s) level, we get the leak! Oestrogens help restore normal blood flow to the tissue and muscles that sustain and regulate the urinary tract. Restoring our body with bioidentical hormones can very easily treat, and even prevent, this common problem. No more sanitary towels needed, or patented medications that cause more problems than they solve, and definitely no need for surgery. Also, interestingly, with age, the majority of women lose their muscle tone in the pelvic floor because of a decline in the production of anabolic hormones. These hormones help keep the muscles strong, so when they are low or deficient, they can hugely contribute to these leakages. Restore your body.

Please take heed: HRT cannot get these results. This was proved by the WHI clinical trial. The authors of the study concluded that "Conjugated equine oestrogen with or without progestin should not be prescribed for the prevention or relief of UI." Also, considering the outcome of elevated risk of heart disease and cancer in this study, it is a 'no-no' for long-term use. Go bioidentical.

HELP! How Do I Stop Vaginal and Urinary Tract Infections?
(A Veritable Workshop in your Vagina)

Well, quite easily, really! Let me explain. Women's vaginal fluids are normally acidic and not without good reason. This acidity makes the vagina more hospitable to a certain type of friendly bacteria called Lactobacillus acidophilus, a bacterium that is also found in yoghurt. Lactobacillus acidophilus thrives in an acidic ambient and also chips in, as it were, by secreting lactic acid. These lactic acid-secreting Lactobacilli in the vagina create a natural barrier against microorganisms that cause disease, the most common of which is E. coli (Escherichia coli). E. coli normally originates in the colon and rectum and, as this area is so close to the vagina and urinary tract in women, is easily transported. Lactobacilli also protect the vagina from yeasts such as Candida albicans (thrush). I suffered from all of these; continual bouts of thrush and forever at the doctor's every other month for antibiotics for urinary tract infections. Once again, I couldn't understand why and, believe it or not, neither could my gynaecologist or GP.

The Reason Why

In menopause, vaginal acidity declines along with oestrogen(s) levels – menopause has got a lot of explaining to do. For this reason the vagina is less hospitable to Lactobacilli and more hospitable to unfriendly, acid-frightened bacteria and yeasts, which find low pH (acidity) injurious to their survival.

As I found out for myself, constant antibiotics only exacerbate the situation. They may kill off the original 'bug' for a time, but they also kill off essential microorganisms that live in the vagina and GI tract and perform many important natural functions. They do nothing to restore a healthy vagina and urinary tract, nor do they help normal acidity of the vagina or the friendly bacteria that once lived there, as bioidentical oestrogens would, which efficiently bring things back into balance. Once again, their aim is to cure the symptom but not the cause. In fact, once the antibiotic is stopped, it will likely encourage further infection, largely due to the fact that the harmless and beneficial Lactobacilli have been wiped out by the antibiotic drug, along with the original infection. (No natural barrier anymore.) Yeasts can now move in easily, which in turn will lead to thrush, which in turn will lead to the need for an antifungal drug. It seems to never finish – you are given your antifungal drug and that seems to put that problem right for the time being but, unless you keep your vagina and urinary tract tip-top clean and bacteria-free, E. coli or some other bad bacteria are likely to return, leading to the vicious cycle of more antibiotics followed by another run of antifungal drugs, and so the story goes on. So now I know why I kept getting urinary tract infections, but I can't help wondering if my gynaecologist and GP have realised yet.

I do not have this problem anymore. I simply restored my body with the oestrogens that were missing. By restoring your body these problems can be prevented and reversed.

A Healthy Heart

Not all hormone replacement regimes are dangerous for women's cardiovascular health – only synthetic ones.

Heart disease is a term used to identify a number of diseases that affect the heart and sometimes the blood vessels. Heart disease or cardiovascular disease includes coronary artery disease, arrhythmia (irregular heartbeat), blocked vessels that may lead to heart attacks or stroke, heart infections and heart defects we are born with. Heart disease is the number one killer in both men and women worldwide.

Women taking oestrogens, along with progesterone, at menopause not only eliminate the menopausal symptoms (hot flushes, mood swings, etc.), they regain their life and the quality of it; they live longer and develop heart disease much more slowly or maybe not at all. They have half the risk of dying from a heart attack than women of the same or similar age who are not taking oestrogens. Also, when supplementing with testosterone along with oestradiol (E2), it lowers our cardiac risk.

Vasodilation and Coronary Blood Flow

A mixture of natural or bioidentical oestrogens and progesterone at balanced and correct ratios promotes healthy vasodilation and coronary blood flow in postmenopausal women. When the heart muscle does not receive a continual supply of blood, feeding it with oxygen and nutrients (a condition known as myocardial ischemia), it could then become severely and permanently damaged. Arteries that get clogged with atherosclerotic plaque may constrict too much or for too long (vasospasm), which may deprive the heart muscle of blood exactly when it may need it most. This can cause heart pain, arrhythmia, heart failure and heart attack. Oestrogens and progesterone are partially in charge of the coronary arteries; they facilitate the dilation and constriction of coronary arteries, making sure the heart muscle receives the blood it needs when required. When there is a decline and our oestrogens and progesterone levels dwindle, our risk of heart disease increases dramatically and eventually becomes the same as a man's. Did you know that there are more women who die of heart attack after menopause than of breast cancer?

When there is an imbalance and oestrogen(s) levels become too high or dominant, their protective qualities reverse. The risk of blood clots and fluid imbalance goes up. This is when natural progesterone used alongside oestradiol (E2) balances out this excess. It is extremely important to keep a balance between these two hormones.

A substance in our blood called fibrinogen increases when our oestrogen(s) levels decrease. This substance is clot-promoting, so in menopause, when our oestrogen(s) levels decline, our fibrinogen can increase and may cause a heart attack. Restoring your body to youthful and optimal levels is the best way to protect yourself.

Not many people (including your doctor) are aware of the above facts and totally blame high cholesterol levels for heart attacks. Not so! Half of all women who die from heart disease have normal cholesterol levels. We will talk more about cholesterol and heart disease later on in the book.

Osteoporosis and Solving the Problem

So, where do we start? Generally, we all know what osteoporosis is and that fragile bones are the crux of the situation, but do we really understand the importance of hormonal involvement? Do we understand that embracing restorative medicine can help resolve and even reverse osteoporosis?

Osteoporosis is a progressive disease and is sometimes called the 'silent disease'. I remember my grandmother. As a child I used to look at her and wonder why she had a hump on her back – now I know it is called a dowager's hump. I used to feel so desperately sorry for her, not only because of her humped, bent-over structure, but also because of her blindness, which was due to age-related macular degeneration. It made me feel so sad, I never wanted to get old. After all, that's what it was, old age. Not for me. She died in an old people's home after she fell and broke her hip. Sad and lonely – how I cried. We are so much luckier today to be able to make a choice. Restorative medicine is that choice.

We all know that bones serve as a reservoir for minerals, especially calcium, that may be needed by other parts of the body. That's why it is important to consume a healthy diet rich in calcium to supply the body with its daily needs, thus avoiding the necessity to raid the bone storage vaults, which would leave the bones deficient in calcium. Bones need calcium for strength, but the process is not as simple as that. Calcium cannot form new bone tissue all on its own. It needs a little help from our friends – these include the major sex hormones oestrogens, progesterone, testosterone and DHEA, as well as parathyroid hormone, vitamin D, magnesium, prostaglandins, growth factor and others, but let's just start with oestrogens and progesterone.

Even though adult bones have stopped growing in length, they still continue to remodel themselves. This remodelling is a normal bodily function; we may not realise that bone is a living tissue, perhaps because of its strength and rigidness, but it is forever renewing and reshaping itself and this is how fractures heal. Remodelling starts when the bone gets broken down by cells called osteoclasts. Osteoclasts work by travelling through the bone tissue searching out older bone cells. When they find these old bone cells, they dissolve them, releasing the bone's calcium and other minerals into the circulation. This is known as bone resorption. As nature would have it, this is where tissue-building cells called osteoblasts step in. Osteoblasts build fresh, new bone tissue by filling in all the little holes that osteoclasts have left behind, by drawing calcium, magnesium and other minerals out of the circulation.

Under normal circumstances, osteoclast and osteoblast live harmoniously together, each balancing the other out, however after menopause, because of the decline in oestrogen(s) levels, osteoclasts begin to run havoc over our bones, literally eating their way through them, creating an increase in bone resorption. It is oestrogen(s) levels that keep the remodelling balance in check by overruling the bone-eating process created by osteoclast activity. Importantly, progesterone is a key factor in rebuilding new bone. With the decline of progesterone just before, during and after menopause the bone-building powers of osteoblasts do not function as before: our little workmen are not able to draw the calcium and other minerals out of the circulation to repair the damage. What this means is that bone health and strength are dependent on a balanced ratio of these two hormones. When our bodily production runs out of oestrogens and progesterone, our bones start to die. When there is an oestrogen(s) deficiency, unrestrained bone resorption literally strips bones of essential calcium and minerals. When there is a progesterone deficiency, new bone cannot form, so cannot replace what has been lost. When both hormones are deficient, as happens in menopause, osteoclast activity (bone-eating process) cannot be rebuilt by osteoblast activity (bone-building process), causing bones to waste away at great speed, and even more so if nutrients like calcium and vitamin D are also deficient. A recent article published in the *New England Journal of Medicine* (July 2012) revealed a protective effect for high-dose vitamin D supplementation against the risk of fracture in older women and men. Vitamin D is required for the absorption of calcium to help make bone.

Testosterone and DHEA are, like progesterone, important bone-builders, and stimulate the formation of new bone in both sexes. Testosterone also makes the bones strong. And amazingly, even melatonin helps prevent bone loss. It signals the production of bone matrix proteins and increases the production of growth hormone. In bone, a matrix is composed of a flexible substance called collagen. Melatonin also blocks osteoclast formation and promotes osteoblast proteins and procollagen production – both these things help in bone-building.

Men also get osteoporosis but this is due to a testosterone deficiency rather than an oestrogen(s) decline. It takes longer for osteoporosis to show up in men because their thicker and denser bones need more time to lose tissue before becoming fragile. Men are at a greater risk, however, of becoming permanently disabled or dying if they break a hip. Believe it or not, a man is more likely to suffer from a fracture related to osteoporosis than prostate cancer.

Women are affected eight times more than men by osteoporosis and our odds of getting it are one in three. We may not even be aware that our body is telling us we are on the way to osteoporosis. Subtle signs such as chronic back pain, or sharp, shooting pains in our back as we bend to pick something up, which may be caused by mini crush fractures in the spine, are warnings. Bone loss presents all these problems. Your posture may be slumped and your stomach may protrude, due to a weakened spine caused by fractures. Take heed, we can protect ourselves, but time is of essence.

Timescale

What we women may not realise is how important it is to take oestrogens and progesterone at the right time in our lives. As I said, osteoporosis is a progressive disease: bone tissue dissipates slowly over many years and with no clear symptoms. Immediately after menopause, some women can have considerable bone loss but generally, osteoporosis doesn't strike for another twenty to thirty years, as the bones have become thinner and weaker. If you have kept your bones strong before menopause through weight-bearing exercises, which maintain both the muscle and bone and keep them healthy and strong, and have a healthy diet, your bones will take longer to thin out and weaken after menopause.

Most women are advised to start taking HRT in their early fifties when their bones are still reasonably strong, but the crazy thing is that our bones need oestrogens and progesterone much more as we reach our seventies and eighties and, of course, by this time we have already been told to stop taking any kind of hormone replacement therapy. Why? Basically, because HRT (synthetic hormones) just ain't safe. But the important thing here is that we need to take these precious hormones for life to keep us strong. So what's the answer? Bioidentical oestrogens and progesterone (along with testosterone) can be taken with no risk to our health. It is possible to reverse bone loss in most women when a complete restorative approach is followed. There is no drug that can do this, neither Fosamax or raloxifene.

Fosamax was designed to inhibit osteoclasts from doing their normal task of breaking down bone, which slows down the loss of BMD (bone mineral density). This does not restore what is missing and has nothing to do with balancing oestrogens and progesterone ratios, or restoring calcium or any other natural bodily requirements. It is a drug that interferes with the natural cycle of bone growth, which cannot be healthy.

Raloxifene is designed to inhibit bone resorption and acts as an oestrogen-like drug. It can cause varying side effects, some not so nice and some very nasty – hot flushes, leg cramps, vision changes – and has been associated with an increased risk of blood clots in the legs and lungs, although these are very rare. Who really wants to take this on when we now have bioidentical hormone replacement therapy?

Nutrients such as calcium (calcium citrate is your best shot), boron, zinc, copper, magnesium, phosphorous, manganese, silicon, strontium, vitamins B6, B12, D and K and folate can certainly help bone health, but are not enough to prevent osteoporosis. We need those precious little, but oh so important, hormones to protect us from becoming chalk.

8. THE DREADED STATIN DRUGS AND CHOLESTEROL

We are nearly at the end of this incredible journey but I am not going to let you go just yet. That would be so unfair, considering I promised to tell you about cholesterol and heart disease. It's an eye-opener.

Cholesterol is the Building Block of Life

I have already mentioned how vital cholesterol is to body function, and its relationship with steroid hormones. Generally today, it is believed that high cholesterol levels are dangerous, but truth be known, to be truly healthy, we need normalised levels of cholesterol in our body, neither too high or too low. This book continually talks about balance, so why stop now? Our body needs balance. Our body is constantly seeking to obtain homeostasis, and works together with our bodily systems through a multiple feedback loop mechanism to achieve this. Our body and mind are very intelligent, and are working at all times to protect us as best they can. When a spanner (monkey wrench) is thrown in the works, 'clink, clank', it messes things up and along comes a myriad of other problems.

The Cholesterol Scare

Cholesterol. Here we go again: you hear the word. What is your immediate thought? Let's play word association for a second. Cholesterol – fear. Cholesterol – shaking in your boots. Cholesterol – bad, cholesterol – the end. High cholesterol – heart attack. There's the supposed link. This little brainwashing technique has come about because of a verbatim syndrome, or as

Dr Dzugan so rightly says, "an ad nauseam setup". This is a hoax that has been going on for over half a century. Manipulation by repetition is the correct term. We have been force-fed it: "Take a statin or two and you'll be OK!" Adverts for cholesterol-lowering drugs (at least in America), and even supplements, along with foods that are low in cholesterol, are thrown at us every day. Cholesterol: bad, bad, bad. "Let's get it out of your body, it will kill you" is what they keep throwing at us. The words 'cholesterol' and 'atherosclerotic plaque' go hand in hand. Diagrams and wall charts, doctors telling us, "Oh, your cholesterol is a little too high, perhaps you should consider taking statins. Let me just write you a prescription, don't want your arteries getting clogged up with cholesterol, do we now?" have brought about this false representation. It is pure manipulation by the statin industry that has caused the cholesterol scare. There are certainly more factors involved in heart attack that need be considered.

Cholesterol has been portrayed as the culprit behind hardening of the arteries (arteriosclerosis) and plaque in the arteries (atherosclerosis); unfortunately we are not getting the full story here. Again, I ask why? It cannot be denied that cholesterol has some involvement in atherosclerotic plaque but it is definitely not the major element. Inflammation, not cholesterol, is a possible culprit in heart disease. You may remember that inflammation increases with age and works against us, becoming chronic rather than transitory as time goes on. What happens in the case of the heart is that toxins and inflammatory by-products are produced that damage and clog the lining of the arteries. Toxins damage our DNA, which increases our risk of cancer, Alzheimer's and significantly increase our risk of heart disease and stroke.

There is an increased risk of heart attack because inflamed arteries are not operating correctly. Nuclear factor kappa beta (NFkB) is a common inducer of chronic inflammation, therefore very dangerous. Age brings with it terrible things, as we know, one of which is an overexpression of this molecule. If you live an unhealthy lifestyle, and are in poor health, you will flick the switch of inflammation on, but if you are in a good state of health the switch of inflammation will be flicked off. In other words, NFkB can work for or against us. It regulates the immune system and inflammation genes. It is the patrolman that looks out for hazards such as free radicals and toxic invaders.

To help NFkB function correctly and avoid inflammation we should try and eliminate excess body fat, reduce stress, get adequate sleep, keep blood sugar levels low so we can avoid diabetes, exercise regularly, *get our hormones balanced* (like I said, this medicine is your greatest defence against cancer and heart attack), not consume too much animal fat, make sure vitamin D levels are optimal, and supplement with omega-3 fish oils, curcumin and antioxidants.

Some of the underlying factors of coronary heart disease, and which also apply to stroke, include high C-reactive protein levels. Basically, this is an inflammation marker, and an important marker for heart attack. High levels of CRP happen when there is inflammation in the body, which is a risk factor for heart disease, diabetes and hypertension. Any doctor can do this simple blood test for you to see how much inflammation you have in your system. A high-sensitivity CRP test is more accurate for measuring cardiovascular disease risk than the standard CRP, as this test is designed to measure inflammation in the body, due to any cause. Also, excess fibrinogen comes into play here – I spoke about this earlier. It is a clot-promoting substance and in menopause, when our oestrogens decrease, fibrinogen levels increase, which may provoke a heart attack. Low testosterone levels, nitric oxide deficit and low EPA and DHA (omega-3 fatty acids) are also underlying factors of coronary heart disease.

Elevated homocysteine levels are another risk factor for developing heart disease. Homocysteine is a common amino acid (one of the building blocks that make up proteins). High levels of homocysteine may be genetic, which is usually due to a defective enzyme (methylenetetrahydrofolate reductase), which breaks down homocysteine. When there is a deficiency of this enzyme the body needs extra folate and we should consider supplementing with it, along with vitamin B6 and B12. Sex hormones have been seen to modulate homocysteine blood levels. A low oestrogen(s) status has also been linked to elevated homocysteine. In menopause oestrogen(s) levels decline, leaving us with elevated homocysteine. We should make sure to get them checked regularly, mainly because elevated homocysteine levels damage the arterial lining, causing them to narrow and become inelastic, which is the condition known as arteriosclerosis. Another important point is that high homocysteine levels lower the production of nitric oxide, which may lead to elevated blood pressure, another risk factor for heart disease. Oh, and one more thing, high homocysteine levels raise triglyceride and cholesterol synthesis.

With elevated lipoprotein(a) levels there is an increased risk of heart attack. Lipoprotein(a) is a small particle that causes inflammation, which can clog our blood vessels. Lipoprotein(a) regulates blood clot formation and decreases blood thinning; when blood becomes too thick there is an increased risk of heart attack and stroke. Although elevated lipoprotein(a) is usually inherited, levels rise naturally after menopause and in diabetics, which increases our risk of heart disease. Some useful information is that statin drugs actually increase lipoprotein(a). People with high lipoprotein(a) levels have a 70% increased risk of developing heart disease over ten years.

For you to get a clear and certainly more truthful picture of this cloud-covered heart attack story, and to enable you to weigh up the pros and the cons for yourselves, let's talk more in depth about statins and the statin industry.

The Spanner in the Works

Statins are a multi-billion dollar industry; it really is big business! And guess what? It seems that everyone over fifty is on these terrible cholesterol-lowering drugs (CLD). (Could there be a hormonal connection?) Again, it's conventional medicine's etiquette of filling up our medicine cabinets;

they really are killing us. In the UK, statin drugs are used even when our total cholesterol levels are ideal. Incredible! Apparently, a study done in 2002, the Heart Protection Study, which involved twenty thousand people, showed that statins appeared to lessen the risk of major cardiovascular problems in everyone. What are they talking about? So, if you are following me, when your doctor prescribes a statin drug for you it is no longer based on cholesterol levels. Whoa, statins are for everyone, like candies from your favourite sweet shop. Or at least, everyone who has a 20% or greater risk of developing CHD (coronary heart disease) over the following ten years, whatever their cholesterol levels may be. How is this risk calculated? Well, this is quite incredible too. It is calculated from charts. Charts based on whether you smoke, your blood pressure, your gender and age, and whether you have diabetes. They do take a look at your cholesterol levels as well though – credit where credit is due. Not that I believe there is any credit due to a statin drug. The mechanism behind statins is to inhibit cholesterol. Can statins stop you from becoming a diabetic, stop you smoking, change your gender or your age? Smoking affects the function of heart and blood vessels, which increases our risk of atherosclerosis but does not raise cholesterol levels. Yes, diabetes does have some influence on cholesterol levels, and yes, diabetics tend to have more cholesterol abnormalities than the rest of the population but this should not be the sole reason for prescribing statins to these people. Just because they have a predisposition to heart attack and stroke does not mean that they necessarily should be prescribed statins. A clear, graceful, fair and humanistic judgement is needed in such cases. Yes, cholesterol levels increase with age, but this is because our hormones decline (I will talk more about this later). And yes, men are at a high risk of heart attack approximately ten years before women of the same age. This would be partially due to a decline in testosterone levels. It is to do with 'pumping potency'. Remember, testosterone improves tissue oxygenation and strengthens and protects the heart by nurturing the cardiac muscle.

Do you think this is a money-making industry or a fair play industry? Has the statin industry taken over? And, to continue, can statins control inflammation? Let me answer that for you. Statins suppress NFkB response, so because of this process appear to work, but remember NFkB can either work for or against us, and by doing so, it messes with our immune system. By suppressing NFkB we inhibit the functionality of our immune system, and when this happens inflammation has the chance to break loose. The fire is blazing, and will get out of control, which can cause cancers and heart disease, among other things. And, for that matter, can statins correct the cause of high cholesterol levels? I think not. Statins work to treat the effect rather than the cause. They do not resolve the problem of high cholesterol, they cover up the cause.

Cholesterol-lowering drugs (CLD) is a blanket term for various medications but statins is the name which is perhaps most well known. Lipitor (atorvastatin), Pravachol (pravastatin), Crestro (rosuvastatin), Mevacor (lovastatin – not licenced for use in the UK), Zocor (simvastatin) and Lescol and Lescol XL (fluvastatin) are all statins. Along with statins there are other CLD groups, which come under the names of cholesterol absorption inhibitors, bile acid sequestrants and fibrates. These groups of agents all follow the same theme, affecting the basic mechanism of cholesterol in a major way. They put a spanner in the works!

How Cholesterol is Inhibited by Statins

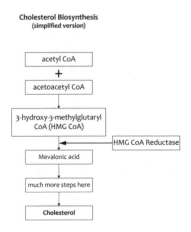

Cholesterol Biosynthesis
(simplified version)

acetyl CoA
+
acetoacetyl CoA

3-hydroxy-3-methylglutaryl
CoA (HMG CoA)

HMG CoA Reductase

Mevalonic acid

much more steps here

Cholesterol

A molecule of cholesterol is primarily synthesised or produced from Acetyl CoA through the reductase pathway, known as 3-hydroxy-3-methylglutaryl CoA (HMG-CoA). HMG-CoA is then acted upon by an enzyme called HMG-CoA reductase, which eventually goes on to create the final product, cholesterol. Statins work by inhibiting the enzyme HMG-CoA reductase, therefore cutting cholesterol production off at its prime. This then goes on to affect the cascade of steroid hormones that are produced from cholesterol. Our hormones, our precious hormones! Those precious, forever-communicative molecules become stymied, muted, blocked; they can no longer instruct. Cholesterol is our most precious molecule, and our most generous. It is indispensable to our health: without it our evolution would be impossible.

Who is Cholesterol?

Before I go any further, let's talk more in depth about who cholesterol is and how it functions within the body, and why we so desperately need it. As I stated earlier, cholesterol is found in all cells of our body, and is important for the routine repair of tissues, suggesting that our body needs it to function correctly. Without cholesterol our cells would be unable to protect themselves from oxidation. In fact, cholesterol is one of the most important molecules in the human body. Cholesterol is the major building block from which cell membranes are made, therefore extremely important to the production of cells. Cholesterol gives the skin the ability to shed water. Cell membranes cover the cells and protect them; being semi-permeable they let things in and out as needed for optimal function. Were a cell not to have this protective layer it would not survive. Again, we need cholesterol in our body for optimal functioning.

The brain produces an interesting amount of cholesterol, in fact 25% is localised within the brain, with most of it present in the myelin. All cholesterol in the brain is a product of local synthesis, since plasma lipoproteins are unable to cross the blood-brain barrier.

So, in essence, all cholesterol in the brain is made in the brain because of this barrier. What is even more interesting is that cholesterol is embedded in the myelin sheath, and our brain and nerve tissue require cholesterol for the formation of the myelin sheath. The myelin sheath is a fatty material made up of 27% cholesterol, 43% phospholipid and 30% protein, and winds around nerve cell axons. So basically, the myelin insulates nerve cells, helps regenerate cut axons and intensifies impulses or electrical signals (messages) throughout our nervous system's circuitry. Many degenerative diseases are associated with an imbalance of cholesterol in the brain, including Alzheimer's disease. Looking at it logically, we should not attack, disturb or inhibit synthesis of this substance, but rather normalise it. When we take statin drugs our brains are in danger. I must stress that every neuron in the brain needs cholesterol to reproduce. Statin drugs inhibit our bodily production of cholesterol, leaving us without the fundamental mechanism to create new and healthy brain cells.

Statin drugs are terrible things; they break the brain and body down. It is not cholesterol we need to be afraid of, but statin drugs themselves. Everyone, at some time, has forgetful moments, or senior moments, the moments I spoke about earlier on in the book. These 'moments' can be rectified by restoring the body with bioidentical hormones, but statin drugs kill our brain. Frightening. They inhibit that major substance called cholesterol which we all need, at normalised levels, in our body and brain to keep them working at optimum. Symptoms caused by statin drugs may begin almost immediately, within weeks of starting this horrific medication, or they may take longer, several years sometimes. My friend's mother found herself confused and disorientated and was unable to move her legs, literally unable to get out of bed, within the first few weeks of taking the medication. Other symptoms can include mild amnesia to severe memory loss, and eventual Alzheimer's. Why are these drugs on the marketplace when they destroy our brain, mangle our thoughts, hurt our family's serenity? The stress on families, seeing our loved ones decline, is a peace-breaker. Dr Dzugan has a safe and effective alternative. Save your brain.

The liver! Yes, the liver is another organ to take a look at. The liver is of major importance in the regulation of cholesterol in the body as it synthesises cholesterol (along with triglycerides), so it can be transported all over the body. The cholesterol that is not needed is transported back to the liver where it is converted into bile salts, which form part of bile, after which it can be eliminated in faeces. Not all of the cholesterol that has been put into bile is excreted out of the body; some is reabsorbed and then processed and reused as needed. Why would the body reuse this cholesterol if it were so bad for our heath?

The liver produces approximately 75% of the body's cholesterol and about 70% of this is used to make bile. Bile is made up of hormones, bile salts, toxins and of course cholesterol. Bile is stored in the gall bladder between meals and is part of our digestive mechanism. The gall bladder is pear-shaped and is situated just below the liver. When food enters the duodenum, a release signal is sent to the gall bladder to squirt bile into the small intestines to help with the digestion and distribution of all lipids (fats), including cholesterol, taken in through diet; not just greasy foods, but healthy, essential fats such as omega-3 fatty acids. Without bile this process could not happen. Nearly all the cholesterol that reaches our gut, about 97%, is absorbed straight back into our bloodstream and sent back to the liver for processing. Bile, of course, has other functions as well, e.g. aiding the absorption of fat-soluble vitamins and dividing up endotoxins to prevent their entry into the bloodstream. Endotoxins are toxins, as the word suggests, or bacteria. They are a part of the cell wall of microorganisms (bacteria).

The reason I am telling you this is to help you understand that we have cholesterol in the body for a reason. Nature did not just give us this substance to make our lives difficult, it gave it to us to help the human skyscraper stand tall and function correctly. Trying to eliminate cholesterol entirely is not the correct way of dealing with things. Like I said, cholesterol is present in all our cells, and two major organs in our body produce the stuff. How come it's so bad then? The story about cholesterol has, somehow, along the way, definitely got mixed up. Manipulation.

The True Story

The true story is that we need to balance cholesterol levels or normalise them for the body to function correctly, not eliminate it or disrupt the production of it. Levels of cholesterol that are too low, as well as levels that are too high, are not good. A host of studies show that low cholesterol concentration increases mortality from haemorrhagic stroke and violent deaths, such as suicide. Having just the right amount is critical to our health. The Honolulu Heart Program is an ongoing study of cardiovascular disease in 8,006 men and began in Hawaii in 1965. Obviously, being a long-term study it is much more beneficial than a short-term study because of the increased data obtained. One of the things that this study showed was that long periods of low cholesterol increased mortality, and that patients who had a lower concentration at a younger age had greater risk of death. This means that young individuals with low concentrations of cholesterol will still have an increase of cholesterol production with age, like any of us, but since cholesterol levels were low to begin with their mortality risk increases compared to another individual who is, let's say, ten years older, with the same cholesterol levels. In other words, it is not good to have cholesterol levels that are too low. Overall, this study showed that it is not a good idea to try and reduce cholesterol levels in the elderly; it cuts their life short. Elderly individuals with the lowest total cholesterol levels have the highest rate of death from coronary heart disease, whereas individuals with elevated total cholesterol levels have a lower risk of coronary heart disease. Blood cholesterol levels rise every ten years until we reach the age of seventy; after that, they stabilise, then start to decline. By the time we reach eighty, there is a significant drop. Is there any need, then, for CLD for the elderly?

Let me recap: cholesterol helps make the coating of our cells, it makes up the bile salts (acids) that help to digest food in the intestines, and it allows the body to make vitamin D and hormones such as pregnenolone, oestrogen and testosterone etc. If our happy friend cholesterol were not around, none of these functions could happen, and we humans would not exist. If cholesterol were not around, we could not produce the correct amounts of steroid hormones and an imbalance would occur.

Cholesterol on its Travels

Cholesterol is oil-based and usually classified as lipid or fat. It is also known as a sterol, which is a combination of a steroid and an alcohol, but it does not behave like alcohol. Cholesterol flows through our bloodstream wrapped in packages made up of protein-covered particles, appropriately named lipoproteins. The reason the body parcels cholesterol up into these packages is because, as I said before, cholesterol is oil-based, but blood is water-based, so they don't mix well. Imagine dropping a few drops of olive oil into water. What happens? The oil droplets float around and form globules, going nowhere, or even somewhere they shouldn't. These packages facilitate the transportation of lipoproteins in the blood so they can be used as needed by the body. Their actual job is to act as carriers for insoluble cholesterol and triglycerides. Triglycerides are commonly known as fats.

There are various types of lipoproteins but the most well-known are HDL (high density lipoprotein), which conventional medicine considers 'good' cholesterol, and LDL (low density lipoprotein), which conventional medicine considers 'bad'. The difference is in their ratio of protein to lipid. The more fat to protein the packages have, the lower the density, and the higher the protein to fat packages, the higher the density. Generally, lipoproteins are made up of proteins, phospholipids, cholesteryl ester, cholesterol and triglycerides. VLDL (very low density lipoprotein) is another carrier which transports a high percentage of triglycerides (TRG) and a smaller percentage of the other components (hence the reason why it is a very low lipoprotein – more fat to protein ratio). VLDL transport TRG from the liver around the body. As this carrier passes through the circulation, the triglycerides component is removed and is either stored as fat or used as fuel. Triglycerides are important players in heart disease, as high levels can increase the risk of cardiovascular problems. A change of lifestyle and the addition of omega 3-fatty acids (fish oils) or preferably krill oils, which contain phospholipid complex that increases absorption, can help lower triglyceride levels.

The lipoproteins LDL and HDL are known as the two major players in the cholesterol story and the formation of atherosclerosis and heart attack. LDL is the primary plasma carrier and delivery service of cholesterol from the liver to the tissues, or parts of the body, that need it at any given time, where it is then absorbed by the cells. Along with being the primary carrier of cholesterol it also accounts for transporting more than half of lipids circulating in the blood. LDL particles are involved in the formation of plaque on the artery walls, as they can deposit cholesterol into the arteries. LDL transports cholesterol both taken from foods and produced by the body.

HDL is made in the intestines and the liver, and its job is opposite to that of LDL. HDL helps remove cholesterol from the artery walls. It acts like a sponge or vacuum cleaner which sucks up excess cholesterol that is not used up by the tissues or cells and takes it back to the liver, where the HDL particle (package) is reassembled and then the cholesterol is either recycled or excreted into the bile.

All the various types of lipoproteins, which I have avoided naming to save confusion, come in varying sizes and transport the aforementioned components, proteins, phospholipids, cholesteryl ester, cholesterol and triglycerides, but carry different percentages of each component. The percentages are dependent on the body's needs. Each carrier has a specific job, and the components that it carries are dependent on what needs to be transported where at a specific time. Your body is talking again – it is organising itself to maintain balance.

So, if we analyse the situation, the outcome is that the two major players in the cholesterol story, LDL (the supposed 'bad' cholesterol) and HDL (the supposed 'good' cholesterol), are not actually cholesterol but transporters of cholesterol. They have been wrongly named – they are carriers and are doing a job: one actually assists the other, trying to maintain balance. There is no 'good' or 'bad' cholesterol, just carriers that are taking their task on. Calling LDL 'bad' is extremely deceptive and goes on to create an irrational fear within the general public; there is a lack of understanding. Everything happens for a reason.

The Rising of Cholesterol

We already know that cholesterol is the manufacturing plant of steroid hormones. But listen to this; it may not have clicked yet – two and two make five, right? Or that's what the statin industry wants us to believe. But we know better: we know it makes four. When there are low levels of steroid hormones in the body, cholesterol levels rise because the body needs to bring hormone levels back up again; in other words, we need a good supply of cholesterol to create more steroid hormones. It only makes sense that it's four and not five, I mean, things add up. The body does things for a reason. It is continually talking and trying to maintain balance – your body understands itself.

Cholesterol and Ageing

We know that a deficiency of steroid hormones (steroidopenia) is a result of ageing, which is, as Dr Dzugan told me, the primary mechanism that leads to hypercholesterolemia (high cholesterol). The approach that he has developed, and clearly explained to me, shows that hypercholesterolemia is due to age-related, enzyme-dependent down regulation (meaning there is a decrease in cellular components – enzymes) of steroid hormone biosynthesis and their interconversions. If you remember, hormones need the help of enzymes to be converted. Enzymes are our middleman. With age they dysfunction, and the hormones we need can no longer be produced adequately. Our middleman has been downgraded from club class to economy. He is going on holiday but he ain't coming back, or at least, not at the same level.

Hypercholesterolemia is a symptom, it is our body at work again, telling us something is wrong. Hypercholesterolemia is a direct result of the age-related decline in hormone production. Our body is trying to regain homeostasis through a feedback loop but cannot manage to achieve this – our body cannot regain balance because of the age-related, enzyme-dependent down regulation. Try as hard as it might, it won't, it cannot happen, unless some intervention takes place. If hormones are restored to youthful levels there will be no need for the overproduction of cholesterol and hey presto (no, this is not magic, it is science!) – no more high cholesterol. When total cholesterol levels are normalised there is no reason for extra production of HDL (which is a sign of improved function), the carrier that transports cholesterol back to the liver. The only reason a high production of cholesterol occurs is because our hormones request more cholesterol so hormones can be produced at adequate or optimal levels. The body has gone into panic mode, as I see it, and is ageing. Dr Dzugan believes elevation of cholesterol is an excellent ageing marker, which defines the time when patients need to start hormone restorative therapy. A similar situation of elevated cholesterol levels happens during pregnancy. The mother needs extra hormones for herself and her baby, so to be able to produce more hormones the body instinctively produces extra cholesterol, by way of the feedback loop mechanism (don't think we need a statin drug there). Cholesterol levels will then be significantly elevated, and if a woman is unable to increase production of cholesterol there will be an increased risk of miscarriage, due to lack of hormone production or an imbalance. You see, the body does everything for a reason. During times of stress, starvation, exercise, childhood growth and when the immune system is responding to injury, disease or tissue repair the body naturally manufactures extra cholesterol; it's the body's natural defence against the damage of such stress.

Nipped in the Bud

Statin drugs nip cholesterol production in the bud. From this, it is quite obvious, then, that hormonal production will decrease. CLDs are linked to altered hormone levels. Basically, low levels of cholesterol means low production of basic hormones. Cholesterol is our building site, our building blocks, without it we cannot build the human skyscraper and keep it standing straight. Statins or cholesterol-lowering drugs are not the answer to avoiding a heart attack; statins only cover up or diminish the symptom of hypercholesterolemia, which does not confront or resolve the underlying cause. Taking a cholesterol-lowering drug is a 'no brainer'. The risks are too high and quality of life is zero. Several studies suggest that reduction of total cholesterol in serum by CLDs is accompanied by a decrease in coronary heart disease (CHD), but not total mortality. Low serum cholesterol has been correlated to poorly understood morbidity. CLDs can cause serious side effects, some of which result in discontinuation or dose reduction. Side effects range from chest pain, weakness, headaches, insomnia, upper respiratory tract infections, severe rhabdomyolysis (the breakdown of skeletal muscle tissue), renal failure, severe fatigue, fibromyalgia-like pain, depression, high cancer risk, suicide, weight gain, diminished libido and erectile dysfunction and, as I already mentioned, they can cause memory loss, brain damage and dementia, and last but by no means least, death – not a good place to be. Some spanner in the works, that is. This definitely indicates the need to find better treatment regimens for cholesterol elevation. Restoring hormonal balance is definitely your best answer.

'A No Brainer – A Death Sentence'

The incident of congestive heart failure has tripled since statins first came onto the marketplace. Statins deplete coenzyme Q10 (CoQ10), which can contribute to heart disease. CoQ10 is our most significant essential nutrient, is located in all of our cells and is responsible for the energy produced by the human body. The heart and the liver have the largest concentrations of CoQ10; these organs require a great deal of energy, and this is why statins, because they inhibit CoQ10, can lead to heart failure. Supplementing with CoQ10 and balancing your hormones is a good idea if you want to keep your heart healthy and beating strongly. Taking statins is not a good idea.

CoQ10 feeds the mitochondria, our energy-generating motor. So what about the mitochondria, then? If statin drugs deplete CoQ10, it is obvious that they then affect mitochondrial energy production. People taking Lipitor, the most well-known of statin drugs, have been seen to have a more than a 50% decrease in CoQ10 serum levels. Along with the heart, every cell and every tissue is dependent on the supply of mitochondrial energy. Without sufficient amounts of CoQ10 our cells lack the appropriate repair mechanism, in other words they cannot mend themselves. CoQ10 plays a highly significant role within the mitochondria, acting as a very potent antioxidant, its protective powers against free radicals being fifty times stronger than vitamin E. Free radicals are responsible for disease, and break the body down, causing cancers and heart disease.

CoQ10 also keeps the cell lining elastic. Statins break down cell walls and have been indicated in a condition called neuropathy, in which a nerve or group of nerves suffer dysfunction, causing pain. Polyneuropathy, pain in more than one nerve, commonly occurs in long-term statin users. Diabetics are often prescribed statins because of their high-risk status of heart attack. Many longstanding diabetics suffer from peripheral neuropathy, which causes a loss of nerve function, numbness, tingling and pain. Your doctor is aware of these side effects, or should be. So, again, is your doctor using fair and humanistic judgment here? It is a pretty big decision, a fine line between what's right or wrong, or what's needed or what is not needed. Myopathy, a muscle-wasting disease that can cause congestive heart failure, is often seen in statin users. Remember, the heart is a muscle. Statins can impair the pumping functions of the heart.

Another outcome associated with CLD use is myositis (inflammation of the muscle) and the deadly rhabdomyolysis.

Rhabdomyolysis is the most severe form of myopathy and is a serious condition which involves the breakdown of skeletal muscle tissue. When this happens there is a release of muscle fibre, called myoglobin, into the bloodstream, which results in myoglobinuria, and blockage and damage of the kidneys. Myoglobinuria is when there are large amounts of myoglobin present in the urine. Small amounts are usually excreted out of the body in this way, but when there is too much myoglobin in the urine, it can affect the filtration mechanism and cause major problems. Myoglobin can also break down into potentially toxic products, which then go on to cause kidney failure and death. Baycol (cerivastatin), a commonly prescribed cholesterol-lowering drug, was taken off the market in August 2001 because of its association with numerous deaths from Rhabdomyolysis. Remember, all statin drugs use the same mechanism: they inhibit the enzyme reductase, HMG-CoA. Deaths from this horrific form of muscle cell breakdown are still being reported.

The thing is, it is not as though these pharmaceutical companies don't know any better. They know very well that statins inhibit CoQ10; they just don't want us to know. 'Knowledge is power', that kind of thing. In 1990, a large pharmaceutical company, Merck, sought and received a patent to combine a statin with up to 1,000 mg of coenzyme Q10, so as to prevent or alleviate cardiomyopathy (you see, they know). Merck has not yet put this product on the market and has not educated our doctors on the importance of supplementing with CoQ10 to offset the dangers of these drugs to the heart. Why have they withheld it from the marketplace? Because they would have to admit that the horrific statin drug was doing some serious damage. As Merck holds the patent, other drug companies cannot form a statin/CoQ10 combination drug. I'm asking, would they really want to anyway?

Statins and Low Libido

Statins kill sex drive. They inhibit cholesterol and therefore mute our hormones, including our sex hormones, testosterone, oestrogens and progesterone. Testosterone is imperative for sex drive in both women and men. Low levels of sex hormones create sexual problems. Men suffer from erectile dysfunction and women lose their sex drive and their sexual feeling is diminished. Wonder why we are never told about this?

Sex is an important part of life. It can save you from divorce for one thing. Wanting to make love, or have sex, with your partner is natural. Sex is instinctive, natural. It is part of life, it is what keeps us relaxed, stress-free, vibrant, content, glowing. Sex is enchanting, breathtaking and calming. Statins kill sex drive. Take all that away and life becomes sad. Take that away and life becomes something of the past. Yes, we can live without sex but life will not be as beautiful, roses won't be as red and violets won't be as blue. It may sound silly but our minds will not be as creative.

Question and Answer Time

I am asking you, as I have asked myself, why would you want to pop a statin drug into your mouth when they don't actually protect us from heart disease, when they have so many side effects that can kill us, when they deprive the body of its sexual pleasure, when they burn our brains out, when they break our body down, when they make life so damn uncomfortable? Why, when there is an alternative that works? Optimisation and restoration of steroid hormones is the answer to optimised cholesterol levels, no side effects included. By optimising our hormones, the effect (high cholesterol) is corrected because the cause (declining hormone levels – panic mode) is responsible for the effect. No more high cholesterol levels. When we optimise our cholesterol levels, at the same time we optimise our body in a total sense. Cholesterol is not the main man in heart disease; we must stop this way of thinking. Inflammation is more of a direct link to heart disease, so the focus should be on the reduction of inflammation, rather than the cutting off of cholesterol.

The underlying cause of inflammation is age. Age provokes 'body breakdown'. With body breakdown there is a loss of regenerative capacity and an accumulation of cellular damage. What happens is that we get a 'seesaw setup' between damage and repair; this can be seen at every level, from the DNA to the cell, organs and the entire body. The speed at which we age depends on the ratio between damage and repair. Repair, rebuild and regenerate (the three Rs) are usually described as anabolic processes. Instead, the damage we experience and accumulate over time is termed catabolic. Hormonal loss, environmental pollution, highly processed foods, ultraviolet radiation, dehydration, stress, obesity and a sedentary lifestyle are all catabolic accelerators. So to explain, the day our catabolic metabolism ratio exceeds our anabolic movement is the day we start seeing and have to deal with inflammation and the other issues I described. Dr Dzugan believes the main reason for atherosclerosis is a dominance of catabolic processes which start after age thirty and slowly increase. The race is on. The answer is to see who will run the fastest for the longest, anabolic or catabolic metabolism? Which one will maintain a greater hold on the ageing process? It is the balance between the anabolic and catabolic processes that needs to be controlled. Cholesterol is way over there, at the other end of the pitch; it is a bystander.

Remember, we need cholesterol (that wonderful, life-giving substance that nature has given us) in our body for it to function at optimum. Sadly, even with all this mounting evidence that cholesterol is actually irrelevant, the general public still seem to want to hang onto this ingrained notion and fear. Very sad.

Hormones play a critical role in damage and repair because they are the most comprehensive messaging machine in the human body. If we restore our hormones we can balance the damaging process, and the race of life will be easier. The 'seesaw' will be tipped in our favour, helping to support the repair function throughout our body and our brain. It is all to do with physiology of the human body. Regenerating our capacity for repair and reducing cellular damage is key to a long and healthy life. Age is a vicious cycle: the older we get, the faster we age because there is more damage and less repair.

Damage, damage and more damage with little or no repair. Restore your body and protect yourself.

It is important to note that restorative medicine's approach also applies to both familial and relative hypercholesterolemia.

CONCLUSION

So here we are, we have arrived at our final destination. You now have an insight into restorative medicine and understand how it works to keep us healthy and, at the same time, give us longevity. You now have an insight into what ageing is really all about. You now know that ageing does not necessarily mean disease. You now know what there is to know. You know that today's medicine, this medicine, the future of medicine, restorative medicine, looks deep inside the body, at each individual molecule, at cellular messengers and intracellular communication, which work together to co-ordinate harmony between our bodily systems, to keep us healthy. You know that it is possible to enjoy our more mature years and actually look forward to them instead of fearing them. And you now know that it is possible to continue to share these years with your loved ones, together with a fully functional body, mind and soul.

My entry into menopause and my sister's bilateral cancer was a big wake-up call for me. It made me question many things. "Life – what's it really all about? Why is there so much cancer, Alzheimer's, heart disease, obesity and general bad health around?" It made me look around and watch the world. What I saw was shocking. I noticed its wild, crazy way of living, its disregard towards the human body, its hectic, frenetic movements, the fast life. I noticed its deterioration, bad eating habits and the buzz of stress that people didn't even know they were enduring, that I didn't even know I was enduring. I learnt to slow down, I learnt to think. I remember sitting down one day in my comfortable office chair and thinking, "OK, so my body is changing; then I need to change." This whole 'changing episode' helped put my life into perspective. The most important thing to me was my health. My energy levels had dropped and I didn't feel as good as I did; I wasn't as dynamic. This uncomfortable situation was beginning to interfere with my life and my health, and I knew it would only get worse. If the doctors I was searching out could not help me, I would have to do it myself. And I did, I found restorative medicine; I changed my way of thinking, which in turn changed my way of life for the better. I learnt to love myself, in the true sense of the word. I learnt that our body is precious; it is what gives us life. Only 20% of disease is inherited and 80% is the environment that we expose our body to. It is what we personally do to our body that counts. I learnt to take care of myself, even more so than I had done previously. I was not going to let age get the better of me. I restored my body and learnt how to deal with stress. We need to look, as I did, deep into our soul and understand who we really are and what we want from life. This is the first step towards change and being healthy.

My personal conclusion, while sitting in that chair, was what is the purpose of life and the purpose of death if we cannot live life to the full and enjoy every moment of it? When we are not truly healthy we cannot enjoy the seasons of life – pain and discomfort take away our pleasures. To die in pain is something I don't want. I want to be able to walk the walk of life and talk the talk of life, until the end. I want to be able to walk in the park, strong and tall, see the colours of the flowers and the green grass, and hear the birds singing clearly. I want to be able to write a book, read a newspaper and breathe the air that is free for all of us to breathe, in optimal health.

When we are young we steam ahead, and quite rightly so, at full blast towards a wonderful and dynamic future, not realising at the time that it cannot go on forever. As we age most of us forget to slow down, until nature tells us to; until our body starts to change direction and show signs of 'breakdown mode'. This book shows you the true pathway to health and gives you the solution to the ravages of ageing that we see every day on the streets.

Entering the world of restorative medicine truly changed my

world. It gave me the tools, the strength and the chance to live the way I wanted to, not the way someone else wanted me to live. It gave me the chance to write this book and tell you that life can be great if we learn to understand it.

Thank you for reading this book. My love to you all, have a long and healthy life!

REFERENCES

Works Cited

Chapter 4

Barette-Connor E, Mosca L, Collins P, et al. Effects of Raloxifen on cardiovascular events and breast cancer in postmenopausal woman. N Engl. J Med. 2006 Jul 13;355(2): 125-37.

Available at http://pi.lilly.com/us/evista-pi.pdf. Eli Lilly and Co. Indianapolis, IN. Accessed February 21, 2014.

Available at http://www.astarzeneca-us.com/pi/Nolvadex.pdf. AstraZeneca Pharmaceutical. Accessed February 21, 2014.

Barette-Connor E, Grady D. Hormone replacement therapy, heart disease, and other considerations. Ann Rev Public Health. 1998;19: 55-72.

Stamper MJ, Colditz GA. Estrogen replacement therapy and coronary heart disease: a quantitative assessment of the epidemiologic evidence. Prev Med;1991;20: 47-63.

Chapter 5

Melamed M, Castan E, Notides AC, Sasson S. Moleculare and kineti basis for the mixed agonist/antagonist activity of estriol. Mol Endocrinol. 1997;11: 1868-78.

Vogel VG, Constantino JP, Wickerman DL. Effects of Tamoxifen and Raloxifen on the risk of developing invasive breast cancer and other disease outcome: The NSABP

Study of Tamoxifen and Raloxifen (STAR) P-2 Trial. JAMA 2006;295: 2727-41.

Ferenczy A, Gelfand M. The biologic significance of cytologic atypoa in progestogen-treated endomerial hyperplasia. Am J Obstet Gynecol. 1989:260: 126-31.

Feldman HA, Goldstein I, Hatzichristou D, et al. The Massachusetts Male Aging Study. J Urol. 1994 Jan;151(1): 54-61.

Schumacher M. Guennoun R, Ghoumari A, et al. Novel perspectives for progesterone HRT, with special reference to the nervous system. Endocr Rev. 2007;28: 387-439.

Yaffe K, Stawaya G, Lieberburg I, Grady D. Estrogen therapy in postmenopausal woman; effects on cognitive function and dementia. JAMA. 1998;279: 688-95.

Morgentaler A. Harvard Medical School. Testesterone and Prostrate Cancer. An Historical Perspective on a Modern Myth. Eur Urol. 2006 Nov;50(5):935-9.

Available at http://www.life-enthusiast.com/dhea-health-and-youth-hormone-a-96.html. Accessed March 3, 2014.

Barrette-Connor E, Khaw KT, Yesn SS. A prospective study of dehydroepiandrosterone sulfate, mortality, and cardiovascular disease. N. England J Med. 1986 Dec;315: 1519-24.

Casson PR, Lindsay MS, Pisarska MD, et al. Dehydroepiandrosterone supplementation augments ovarian stimulation in poor responders: a case series. Hum Reprod. 2000;Oct15(10): 2129-32.

The biological role of Dehyrdoepiandrosterone (DHEA). Berlin, New York. Walter de Gruyter. 1990; pp.107-130. (The Super Hormone Promise by William Regelson.)

Bloch M, Schmidt PJ, Danaceau MA, et al. Dehydroepiandrosterone treatment of midlife dysthymia. Biol Psychiatry.1999 Jun 15;45(12): 1533-41.

Osuji IJ, Vera-Bolonos E, Carmody TJ, et al. Pregnenolone for cognition and mood in dual diagnosis patients. Psychiatry Res. 2010 Jul 30;178(2): 309-12.

Sanchez-Barcelo EJ, Cos S, Fernandez R, Mediavilla MD. Melatonin and mammary cancer: a short review. Endocr Realt Cancer. 2003 Jun;10(2): 153-9.

Cuzzocrea S, Reiter RJ. Pharmacological actions of melatonin in acute and chronic inflammation. Curr Top Med Chem. 2002 Feb;2(2): 153-65.

Stetinova V, Smetanovà L, Grossman V, Anzebacher P. In vitro and in vivo assessment of the antioxidant activity of melatonin and related indole derivative. Gen Physiol Biophys. 2002 June 21;(2): 153-62.

Reiter RJ, Tan DX, Paredes SD, Funtes-Broto L. Beneficial effects of melatonin in cardiovascular disease. Ann Med. 2010 May 6;42(4): 276-85.

Sofic E, Rimpapa Z, Kundurovic Z, et al. Antioxidant capacity of the neurohormone melatonin. J Neural Transm. 2005;112: 349-58.

Reiter RJ, Parades SD, Korkmaz A, et al. Melatonin combats molecular terrorism at the mitochondrial levels. Interdiscip Toxicol. 2008 Sep;1(2)137-49.

Scrinivasan V, Pandi-Perumel SR, Cardinali DP, et al. Melatonin in Alzheimer's disease and other neurodegenerative disorders. Behav Brain Funct. 2006 May 4;2: 15.

Acuna-Castroviejo D, Escames G, Leòn J, et al. Mitochondrial regulation by melatonin and its metabolites. Adv. Exp Med Biol 2003;537: 549-57.

Yi C, Pan X, Yan H, et al. Effects of melatonin in age-related macular degeneration. Ann NY Acad Sci. 2005 Dec;1057: 384-92.

Massoudi M, Meilahn EN, Orchard TJ, et al. Prevalence of thyroid antibodies among healthy middle aged woman. Findings from the thyroid study in healthy woman. Ann Epidemiol. 1995 May;5(3): 229-33.

Lange U, Boss B, Teichmann J, et al. Thyroid disorders in female patients with ankylosing spondylitis. Eur Jour Med Res. 1999;4(11): 468-74.

Hak E, Huibert AP, Visser TJ, et al. Subclinical hypothyroidism is an independent risk factor for atherosclerosis and myocardial infarction in elderly woman: The Rotterdam Study. Ann Int Med, 15 Feb 2000:132(4): 270-78.

Brownstein D. Iodine: Why You Need It. Why You Can't Live Without It. 2004; West Bloomfield, MI: Medical Alternative Press, 11.

Available at http://www.newsmaxhealth.com/DrBrownstein/iodine-pregnance-IQADHA/2014/10/22/id/548448.

Nils Paulmann, Maik Grohman, Jorg-Peter Voigt, et al. Intracellular seratonin modulates insulin secretion from pancreatic B-Cells by Pr. Published October 27, 2009. DOI:10.1371/journal.pbio.1000229.

Mantozoros CS, Georgiadis EI, Evangelopoulou K, et al. Dehydropiandrosterone sulfate and testesterone are independently associated with body fat distribution in menopausal woman. Epidemiology Vol.7, No5 (Sep,1996), pp. 513-515.

JE Nestler, MA McClanachan, JN Clore, Blackard WG. Insulin inhibits adrenal 17- 20-lyase activity in man. J Clin Endocrinol Met. 1992;74(2): 362-7.

Nestler JE, Strauss JF. Insulin as an effector of human ovarian and adrenal steroid metabolism. Endocrinol Met Clin North Am. 1991 Dec; 20(4): 807-23.

Colacurci N, Zavone R, Mollo A, et al. Effects of hormone replacement therapy on glucose metabolism. Panminerva Med. 1998 Mar; 40(1): 18-21.

Available at http://ghr.nim.nih.gov/handbook/LifeExtension. Accessed Feb 2, 2014.

Cabarcas SM, Hurt EM, Farrar WL. Defining the molecular nexus of cancer, type 2 diabetes and cardiovascular disease. Curr Mol Med, 2010 Nov; 10(8): 744-55.

Crane PK, Walker R, Hubbard RA, et al. Glucose levels and risk of dementia. N. Engl J Med. 2013 Aug 8; 369(6): 540-8.

Available at http://cchrint.org/2013/08/26/sharp-rise-in-uk-women-poisoned-by-antidepressants. Accessed March 3, 2014.

Luboshitzky R. Endocrine activity during sleep. J. Pediatr Endocrinol Metab, 2000 Jan; 13(1) 223-50.

Thorn L, Hucklebridge F, Esgate A, et al. The effects of down stimulation on the cortisol response to awakening in healthy participants. Psychoneurendocrinology. 2004 Aug; 29(7): 925-30.

Boguslawa Baranowska, Ewa Wolinska-Witort Bik, Agnieszka Baranowska-Bik et al. Neurobiology of Aging. 2008 August; 29(8): 1283.

Zeitz B, Hrach S, Scholmerich J, Straub RH. Differential age-related changes of hypothalamus-pituitary-adrenal axis hormones in healthy women and men – role of interleukin 6. Exp Clin Endocrinol Diabetes. 2001; 109(2): 93-101.

Eigh E, Lindqvist Astot A, Fagerlund M, et al. Cognitive dysfunction, hippocampal atrophy and glucocorticoid feedback in Alzheimer's disease. Biol Psychiatry. 2006 Jan; 15:59(2): 155-61.

De Battista C, Belanoff J. C-1073 (mifepristone) in the adjunctive treatment of Alzheimer's disease. Curr Alzheimer's Res. 2005 Apr; 2(2): 125-9.

Belanoff JK, Jurik J, Schatzberg LD, et al. Slowing the progression of cognitive decline in Alzheimer's disease using mifepristone. J Mol Neurosci. 2002 Aug–Oct; 19(1–2): 201-6.

Epel ES, McEwan B, Seeman T, et al. Stress and body shape: stress induced cortisol secretion is consistently greater among woman with central fat. Psychosom Med. 2000 Sep–Oct; 62(5): 623-32.

Villareal DT, Holloszy JO. Effect of DHEA on abdominal fat and insulin action in elderly woman and men: randomized controlled trial. JAMA. 2004 Nov 10; 292(18): 2243-8.

Yong HA, Gallagher P, Porter RJ. Elevation of cortisol-dehydroepiandrosterone ratio in drug-free depressed patients. Am J Psychiatry. 2002 Jul; 159(7): 1237-9.

Goodyer IM, Herbert J, Tamplin A. Psychoendocrine antecedents of persistent first-episode major depression in adolescents: a community-based longitudinal enquiry. Psychol Med. 2003 May; 33(4): 601-10.

Van Niekerk JK, Huppert FA, Herbert J. Salivary cortisol and DHEA: association with measures of cognition and well-being in normal older men, and effects of three months of DHEA supplementation. Psychoneuroendocrinology. 2001 Aug; 26(6): 591-612.

Young AH. Cortisol in mood disorders. Stress. 2004 Dec; 7(4): 205-8.

Arnaldi G, Mancini T, Polenta B, Boscaro M. Cardiovascular risk in Cushing's syndrome. Pituitary. 2004; 7(4): 253-6.

De Leo M, Pibonello R, Auriemma RS, et al. Cardiovascular Disease in Cushing's Syndrome: Heart Versus Vasculature. Neuroendocrinology. 2010; 92 (Suppl 1): 50-4.

Holick MF. Vitamin D: evolutionary, physiological and health perspectives. Curr Drug Targets. 2011 Jan; 12(1): 4-18.

Wacker M, Holick MF. Vitamin D – effects on skeletal and extra skeletal health and the need for supplementation. Nutrients. 2013 Jan; 10; 111-48.

Adam and Hollis. Vitamin D Synthesis, Metabolism, and Clinical Measurements. In Coe and Favus, des. Disorders of Bone and Mineral, Philadelphia: Lippencott, Williams and Wilkins (2002) p. 159.

Pliz S, Tomashcitz A, Marz W, et al. Vitamin D, cardiovascular disease and mortality. Clin Endocrinol (Oxf). 2011 Nov; 75(5): 575-84.

Welsh J. Cellular and molecular effects of vitamin D on carcinogenesis. Arch Biochem Biophys. 2012 Jul 1; 523(1): 107-14.

Krishanan AV, Swami S, Feldman D. The potential therapeutic benefits of vitamin D in the treatment of oestrogen receptor positive breast cancer. Steroids. 2012 Sept; 77(11): 1107-12.

Annwiler C, Rolland Y, Schott AM, et al. Higher vitamin D dietary intake is associated with lower risk of Alzheimer's disease: a 7-year follow up. J Gerontol A Biol Sci Med Sci. 2012 Nov; 67(11): 1205-11.

Lehmann DJ, Refsum H, Warden DR, et al. The Vitamin D receptor gene associated with Alzheimer's disease. Neurosci Lett. 2011 Oct 24; 504(2): 79-82.

Dickens AP, Lang IA, Langa KM, et al. Vitamin D, cognitive dysfunction and dementia in older adults. CNS Drugs. 2011 Aug; 25(8): 629-39.

Holick MF. Vitamin D: a d-lightful solution for health. J Investig Med. 2011 Aug; 59(6): 872-80.

Chapter 7

Grosman N. Study on hyaluronic acid-protein complex, the molecular size of hyaluronic acid and the exchangeability of chloride in the skin of mice before and after oestrogen treatment. Acta Pharmacol Toxicol (Copenh). 1973;33(3): 201-8.

Grosman N, Hvidberg, E, Schou, J. The effect of oestrogen treatment on the acid mucopolysacchride pattern in K skin of mice. Acta Pharmacol Toxicol (Copenh). 1971;30(5): 458-64.

Schmidt JB, Binder M, Demschick G, et al. Treatment of skin ageing with topical estrogens. Int J Dermatol. 1996 Sep;35(9): 669-74.

Sherwin B. Estrogen effects on cognition in menopausal women. Neurology. 1997,May;48(5 Suppl.7): S21-6.

McEwan BS, Wooley CS. Estradiol and progesterone regulate neuronal structure and synaptic connectivity in adult as well as developing brain. Exp Gerontol. 1994;29(3-4): 431-6.

Wooley CS, McEwan BS. Roles of estradiol and progesterone in regulation of hippocampal dendritic spine density during estrous cycle in rat. J Comp Neurol. 1993 Oct 8; 336(2): 293-306.

Henderson VW, Watt L, Buckwalter JG. Cognitive skills associated with oestrogen replacement with Alzheimer's disease. Psychoneuroendocrinol. 1996 May; 21(4): 421-30.

Henderson VW. Estrogen, cognition and women's risk of Alzheimer's disease. Am J Med. 1997 Sep 22; 103(3A): 11S–18S.

Weiland NG. Estradiol selectively regulates agonist binding sites on the N-methyl-D-aspartate receptor complex in the CA1 region of the hippocampus. Endocrinology. 1992 Aug; 131(2): 662-8.

Adler GK, Manfredsdottir VF, Creskoff KW, et al. Neuroendocrine abnormalities in fibromyalgia. Curr Pain Headache Rep. 2002 Aug; 6(4): 289-98.

Rohr UD, Herold J. Melatonin deficiencies in women. Maturitas. 2002 Apr 15; 41(Suppl 1): S85-104.

Chung N, Cho SY, Choi DH, et al. STATT: a titrate-to-goal study of simvastatin in Asian patients with coronary heart disease. Simvastatin treats Asians to target. Clin Ther. 2001 Jun; 23(6): 858-70.

Chapter 8

Benjamin J Ansell, MD, FACC. C-reactive protein: a new tool for evaluating cardiovascular disease risk prediction. HCP. 2007 Dec 10.

Refsum H, Ueland PM, Nygard O, Vollset SE. Homocysteine and cardiovascular disease. Ann Rev Med 1998; 49: 31-62.

Stern LL, Rosenberg IH, Selhub J. Conversion of 5-formyltetrahydrofolic acid to 5-methyltetrahydrofolic acid is unimpaired in folate-adequate persons homozygous for the C677T mutation in the methylenetetrahydrofolate reductase gene. J Nutr. 2000 Sep; 30(9) 2238-42.

Dose-dependent effects of folic acid on blood concentrations of homocysteine: a meta-analysis of the randomized trials.

Am J Clin Nutr, 2005 Oct; 82(4): 806-12. Homocysteine Lowering Trialists' Collaboration.

Stork S, Baumann K, Von Schacky C, Angerer P. The effect of 17 beta-estradiol on MCP-1serum levels in postmenopausal women. Cardiovascular Research. 2002 Feb 15; 53(3): 642-9.

Hak AE, Polderman KH, Westendorp IC, et al. Increased plasma homocysteine after menopause. Atherosclerosis 2000 Mar; 149/(1): 163-8.

Ravnskov U. The Cholesterol Myths. Washington: New Trends Publishing, 2000; ISBN 0-9670897-0-0.

Law MR, Thompson SG, Wald NJ. Assessing possible hazards of reducing serum cholesterol. BMJ. 1994 Feb 5; 308(6925): 373-9.

Hawthon K., Cowen P., Owens D. et al. Low serum cholesterol and suicide. Br J Psychiatry. 1993 June; 162: 818-25.

Law MR, Wald NL, Thompson SG. By how much and how quickly does reduction in serum cholesterol concentration lower risk of ischaemic heart disease? BMJ 1994 Feb 5; 308(6925): 367-72.

Schatz IJ, Masaki K, Yano K, et al. Cholesterol and all-cause mortality in elderly people from the Honolulu Heart Program: a cohort study. Lancet. 2001 Aug 4; 358(9279): 351-5.

Smolarczyk R, Romejko E, Wojcicka-Jagodzinska J, et al. Lipid metabolism in women with threatened abortion. Ginekol Pol. 1996 Oct; 67(10): 481-7.

Papassotiropoulos A, Hawellek B, Frahnert C, et al. The risk of acute suicidality in psychiatric inpatients increases with low plasma cholesterol. Pharmacopsychiatry. 1999; 32(1): 1-4.

Gould AL, Rossouw JE, Santenello NC, et al. Cholesterol reduction yields clinical benefit. A new look at old data. Circulation 1995; 91(8): 2274–82.

Muldoon MF, Ryan CM, Flory JD, Manuck SB. Effects of simvastatin on cognitive functioning. Presented at the American Heart Association Scientific Sessions. Chicago, IL, USA; 2002, Nov: 17-20.

King DS, Wilburn AJ, Wofford MR, et al. Cognitive impairment associated with atorvastatin and simvastatin. Pharmacotherapy. 2003 Dec; 23(12): 1663-7.

Gaist D, Garcia Rodriguez LA, Huerta C, et al. Are users of lipid-lowering drugs at increased risk of peripheral neuropathy? Eur J Clin Pharmacol. 2001 Mar; 56(12): 931-3.

Jacobson TA. Clinical context; current concepts of coronary heart disease management. Am J Med. 2001 Apr 16; 110 supple 6A: 3S-11S.

Chung N, Cho SY, Choi DH, et al. STATT: a titrate-to-goal study of simvastatin in Asian patients with coronary heart disease. Simvastatin Treats Asians to Target. Clin Ther. 2001 June; 23(6): 858-70.

Newman TB, Hulley SB. Carcinogenicity of lipid-lowering drugs. JAMA 1996; 275(1): 55-60.

Black DM, Bakker-Arkema RG, Nawrocki JW. An overview of the clinical safety profile of atorvastatin (Lipitor), a new HMG-CoA reductase inhibitor. Arch Intern Med 1998; 158(6): 577-84.

Available at http://amma.org./mon62.html. Accessed February 12 2014.

Silver MA, Langsjoen PH, Szabo S, et al. Statin Cardiomyopathy? A potential role for Co-Enzyme

Q10 therapy for statin-induced changes in diastolic LV performance: description of a clinical protocol. Biofactors. 2003; 18(1-4): 125-7.

Chronic fatigue, aging, mitochondrial function and nutritional supplements. The Townsend Letter, 2003.

Gaist D, Jeppesen U, Andersen M, et al. Statins and the risk of polyneuropathy: a case-control study. Neurology 2002 May 14; 58(9): 1333-7.

Phillip PS, Haas RH, Bannykh S, et al. Statin-associated myopathy with normal creatine kinase levels. Ann Int Med 2002 Oct 1; 137(7): 581-5.

Chang JT, Staffa JA, Parks M, Green L. Rhabdomyolysis with HMG-CoA reductase inhibitors and gemfibrozil combination therapy. Pharmacoepidemiol Drug Saf. 2004 Jul; 13(7): 417-26.

Scheen AJ. Fatal rhabdomyolysis caused by cerivastatin. Rev Med Liege. 2001 Aug; 56(8): 592-4.

INDEX

Introductory Note
When the text is within a diagram, the number span is in bold.
Eg, adrenal cortex **33**-4